Test-Tube Conception

Test-Tube Conception:

A Blend of Love and Science

BY

E. Peter Volpe

WITH ILLUSTRATIONS BY
Philip Mattes

MERCER
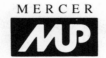

ISBN 0-86554-287-2 (casebound)   MUP/H257
ISBN 0-86554-291-0 (perfectbound)   MUP/P50

Test-Tube Conception:
A Blend of Love and Science
Copyright © 1987
Mercer University Press, Macon GA 31207

The paper used in this publication meets
the minimum requirements of American National Standard
for Information Sciences—Permanence of Paper
for Printed Library Materials, ANSI Z39.48-1984.

Library of Congress Cataloging-in-Publication Data
Volpe, E. Peter (Erminio Peter)
Test-tube conception.

Includes bibliographical references and index.
1. Fertilization in vitro, Human. I. Title.
[DNLM: 1. Fertilization in vitro—popular works.
WQ 150 V931t]
RG135.V64 1987   618.1'78'059   87-22061
ISBN 0-86554-287-2 (alk. paper)
ISBN 0-86554-291-0 (pbk. : alk. paper)

Contents

List of Illustrations

PREFACE

A new page in medical history was written when the world's first "test-tube" baby was born in England in 1978. The baby was originally conceived outside her mother's body in a laboratory dish. This spectacular technique of *in vitro* fertilization—wherein a woman's egg is fertilized outside her body, grown for a few days in culture, and then implanted in her womb—has emerged in a very few years from a scientific curiosity to an almost standard treatment for several common causes of infertility. Some two thousand babies have been born worldwide by this procedure, most of them in England, Australia, and the United States.

The novel procedure that astonished an unsuspecting society on that occasion has since been modified and extended in ways undreamed of by even the most imaginative person. Embryos are being frozen to be thawed later and implanted in a receptive womb. Mixtures of egg and sperm are being injected into the female reproductive system to undergo fertilization there. An embryo can be recovered from one woman by flushing the uterine cavity, and the embryo can then be transferred to another woman. The prospect of remedying a genetic disorder by replacing the faulty gene in the early embryo with the normal gene is within sight.

The newer capabilities have precipitated sharp ethical and legal debate. The relentless medical advances are viewed by some thoughtful observers as a continual assault on the natural biological basis of the family. The accusers see humankind as being treated irreverently as animal husbandry. Humanity, they warn, is rapidly moving toward merchandizing babies just like any other consumer product. But while technology can replace the sex act, it can never replace the love of infertile parents toward a long-awaited child who otherwise would never have been conceived.

Few events are more illustrative of the rapidity and direction of change in our times than the impact of medical knowledge and technology on human life. Progress in medical research has occurred too rapidly to permit the average person to digest the rush of recent discoveries. Much of the new information appears in technical journals not readily accessible to, nor easily understood by, the general reader. Accordingly, this book has been prepared for the interested layperson who is trained neither in science or medicine. My purpose has been to place the facts before the public as simply and responsibly as possible. I have concentrated on the scientific and medical aspects of *in vitro* fertilization. This book considers the historical background and the different approaches to overcoming infertility, the risks involved for the mother and child, and the future promises and threats. I have not avoided the ethical and legal issues, but the views presented are those of intensely interested observer and not as an expert.

Many colleagues at the Medical School of Mercer University contributed to this book in a variety of ways, but some deserve to be singled out for special appreciation. My research associate, Wilma Parrish, once again provided valuable assistance in the seemingly endless details that are involved in the preparation of a book. George Bernard, Lucy Andrews, and Meredith Pratt read and commented insightfully on various chapters. Very gratefully, I thank Ginger Sanders for cheerfully typing the manuscript on a word processor. The drawings, many of them original, are the accomplished work of Philip Mattes, who chose to serve his internship as a medical artist at the Mercer Medical School, for which I am deeply appreciative. Finally, for reasons they alone will understand, I thank my wife, Carolyn, and my three children, Laurie, Lisa, and John.

E. Peter Volpe
Professor of Basic Medical Sciences
Mercer University School of Medicine
Winter 1987

Chapter 1

Tempest in a Test Tube

On the 25th day of July 1978, bold headlines in Britain announced that a thirty-year-old woman in a northern English mill town had given birth to a healthy baby girl who had begun life as a fertilized egg in a culture dish in a medical laboratory. In journalistic vernacular, the world was said to have witnessed its first "test-tube" baby. It seemed as if an ancient prophetic legend of creation of human life in a bubbly glass vial had become a reality. There was, however, no such dazzling alchemy. The test-tube baby was *not* nurtured in a glass womb, completely devoid of any contact with the mother. Indeed, the infant spent only a very brief portion of its nine-months' existence outside the womb of the mother.

The thirty-year-old mother was Lesley Brown, who had tried in vain for nine years to have a child. All therapeutic measures had failed to correct an obstruction in her fallopian tubes, which made the tubes inaccessible to any eggs released by the ovaries. She and her husband John finally placed their faltering hopes on a newly emerging medical measure designed to circumvent the irreparably blocked fallopian tubes. The pioneering procedure was developed by two scientists—Patrick Steptoe, a highly respected surgeon at a hospital in Oldham, England and his longtime Cambridge University colleague, Robert G. Edwards, a well-known reproductive physiologist.

Although separated from each other by 180 miles, the two scientists collaborated for a ten-year period to bring to completion a technique that ultimately led to Mrs. Brown's long-awaited pregnancy.[1] The British team removed an egg surgically from Mrs. Brown's ovary, shortly before it would have been released naturally. The egg was deposited in a round culture dish (not a test tube!) and exposed several hours later to a suspension of sperm (figure 1). Technically, the egg was fertilized *in vitro* (literally, "in glass"). The embryo was grown in culture for a few days and then placed in Mrs. Brown's uterus. Slightly less than nine months later, Mrs. Brown gave birth during a forty-five minute caesarean operation to a five-pound, twelve-ounce girl, named Louise Joy Brown.

The birth of the first child conceived outside the mother's body caught unprepared a society that seems to be threatened by every novel scientific advance. The accomplishment brought forth a mix of conflicting emotional outpourings, ranging from whimsical stories to hostile outcries. The humorist Art Buchwald wrote his usual tongue-in-cheek newspaper column in which he advocated a ban on glass test tubes to prevent their use in manufacturing babies.[2] Theologians sounded warnings about the disturbing moral overtones of such an "unnatural" act. Philosophers were astir with declarations that a moratorium is necessary on ill-conceived experiments that defile nature. The new reproductive technologies have continued to this day to arouse lively debate.

In vitro fertilization holds out the promise of a long-awaited child to many infertile couples. In industrialized nations, problems of infertility strike one out of eight women of childbearing age. Only in recent years have physicians fully appreciated that the fallopian tubes are hopelessly blocked in a large number of infertile women.[3] In the United Kingdom and

---

[1]The accomplishments of Edwards and Steptoe are even more remarkable in that they largely worked independently, at Cambridge University and Kershaw's Hospital in Oldham, respectively. Funds to support the work were not freely available, laboratory space and equipment were sparse, and scant encouragement was received from other colleagues. In fact, each step of the study over the ten-year period was accompanied by a storm of criticism. See R. G. Edwards and P. C. Steptoe, *A Matter of Life* (New York: William Morrow and Company, Inc., 1980) and R. G. Edwards and J. M. Purdy, *Human Conception In Vitro* (London: Academic Press, 1982).

[2]A. Buchwald, "The Right to Chemical Life," *Washington Post,* 13 August 1978.

[3]The rising infertility among young women in their early twenties is alarming. The rate of infertility has tripled in the past two decades as a consequence of an increased incidence of venereal disease with its attendant increase in pelvic inflammatory disease, as well as tubal disease related to the widespread use of intrauterine devices.

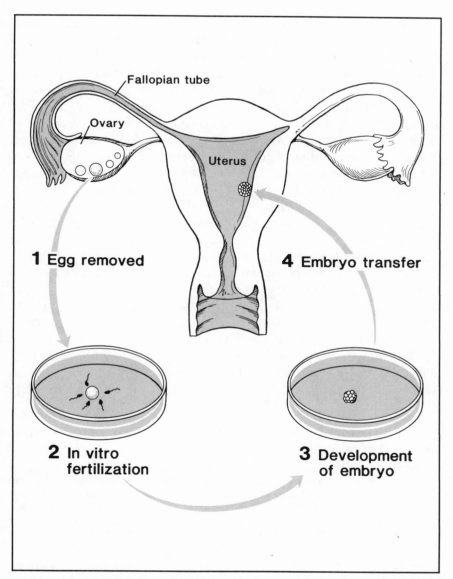

The Technique of *in Vitro* Fertilization **Figure 1**

The egg is removed from the ovary, fertilized in a culture dish, grown in culture to the sixteen-cell stage, and then transferred to the woman's uterus.

the United States, some 700,000 women are infertile because of irreparable lesions in their tubes. It was against this background that Steptoe and Edwards undertook their painstaking study. In the late 1960s, Edwards sought the means of extracting a ripe egg directly from the ovary just prior to its release. Steptoe suggested that they modify a surgical technique called *laparoscopy* to recover the preovulatory egg (figure 2). A clear view of the ovary is obtained with a slender illuminated telescope-like instrument, or laparoscope, which is inserted through a small incision made in the navel. The viewing device illuminates the ovary, enabling the surgeon to examine the surface of the organ. The rounded follicle (containing the ripe egg) is readily detectable on the surface of the ovary as a thin-walled pink swelling. A specially designed hypodermic needle is then passed through a second incision in the abdomen, and the contents of the bulging follicle are aspirated. The entire laparoscopic search and retrieval of the egg can be accomplished in less than two minutes.[4]

Following the identification of the egg in the follicular aspirate taken from Mrs. Brown, the egg was washed in a chemically balanced solution and subsequently deposited in a suspension of the husband's sperm.[5] In addition to the customary practice of examining the semen microscopically to assess sperm motility and morphology, the semen was analyzed for the presence of harmful bacteria. Appropriate antibiotic agents were used to destroy any noxious bacteria.[6] Approximately 18 hours after insemination, the fertilized egg was placed in a growth medium. The early

---

[4]P. C. Steptoe and R. G. Edwards, "Laparoscopic Recovery of Preovulatory Human Oocytes After Priming of Ovaries with Gonadotropins," *Lancet* 1 (1970): 683-89.

[5]Researchers had earlier observed that a human egg has the capacity to divide in an artificial medium even when it had not been penetrated by a sperm cell. Accordingly, the occurrence of fertilization has to be verified by several morphologic criteria, the most prominent of which is the presence of two pronuclei within the egg—the maternal nuclear contribution and the paternal nuclear contribution. See R. G. Edwards, B. D. Bavister and P. C. Steptoe, "Early Stages of Fertilization *in Vitro* of Human Oocytes Matured *in Vitro*," *Nature* 221 (1969): 632-35.

[6]Certain pathogenic bacteria seem to thrive in the semen, particularly in males with abnormal sperm counts. In the absence of antibiotic treatment, the bacteria in the semen can produce infection in the developing embryo. Incredibly, many bacteria in semen can survive freezing in liquid nitrogen, which means that the same stringent laboratory tests must be applied to frozen donor semen. See M. P. McGowan, H. W. G. Baker, D. M. Dretser, and G. Kovacs, "The Incidence of Non-Specific Infection in the Semen in Fertile and Sub-Fertile Males," *International Journal of Andrology* 4 (1981): 657-62.

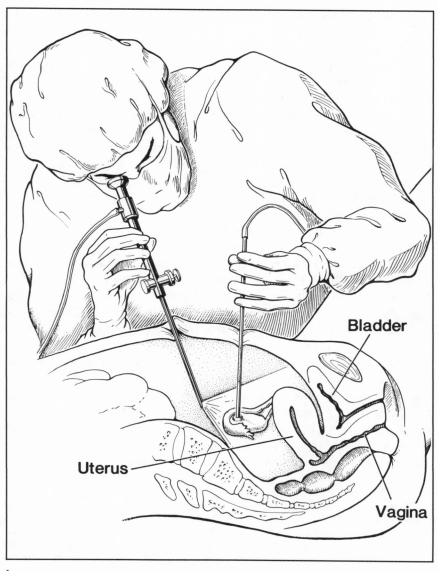

Laparoscopy

Figure 2

A technique for performing various abdominal operations, including the removal of a ripe egg from a woman's ovary.

development of the embryo in culture was observed to follow an orderly, normal pattern. The placement of the embryo in Mrs. Brown's uterus was accomplished without anesthesia and with minimal discomfort to the patient. The embryo, riding in a drop of culture solution, was placed inside a thin tube (cannula) and passed through the cervical canal into the uterus.[7] Mrs. Brown was asked to rest quietly for the next ten hours.

Normally, it takes the fertilized egg nearly a week to find its way into the wall of the uterus (figure 3). Four or five days are spent journeying through the fallopian tube, during which time the egg has divided several times. The successive divisions of the egg are referred to as cleavages. After several cleavages, the embryo—no longer an egg—consists of a solid ball of cells resembling a small mulberry. The embryo floats free in the uterine cavity for two or three days before invading and burrowing into the uterine wall. At the time of implantation, the embryo resembles a hollow sphere and is called a *blastocyst* (figure 4).

Proficiency in growing the human embryo in laboratory culture was achieved only after a prodigious amount of laborious experimental work. In September 1970, Edwards and his co-workers announced in the English journal *Nature* that several *in vitro* fertilized eggs developed normally as far as the sixteen-cell stage.[8] This was followed by a published report in the January 1971 issue of *Nature* that the human embryo could be cultured to the blastocyst stage, at which point it would naturally implant itself in the uterus.[9] Initially, it was anticipated that the best outcome would be attained if the *in vitro* embryos were transferred at the blastocyst stage. However, it was unexpectedly found that the highest proportion of pregnancies occurred when the embryos were transferred at the sixteen-cell stage. Apparently the sixteen-cell stage is synchrony with the hormonal changes that prepare the uterus to receive the embryo.

---

[7]In the numerous trials, the embryos were implanted in the uteri of women at varying times of the 24-hour day. Surprisingly, all successful pregnancies ensued when the embryos were inserted during the late evening. Since this phenomenon may represent an important instance of a biological rhythm in humans, Steptoe and Edwards invariably carried out the implantation only during the evening hours, and not during morning or afternoon hours.

[8]R. G. Steptoe, P. C. Steptoe, and J. M. Purdy. "Fertilization and Cleavage *in Vitro* of Preovulatory Human Oocytes," *Nature* 227 (1970): 1307-1309.

[9]P. C. Steptoe, R. G. Edwards, and J. M. Purdy, "Human Blastocysts Grown in Culture," *Nature* 229 (1971): 132-33.

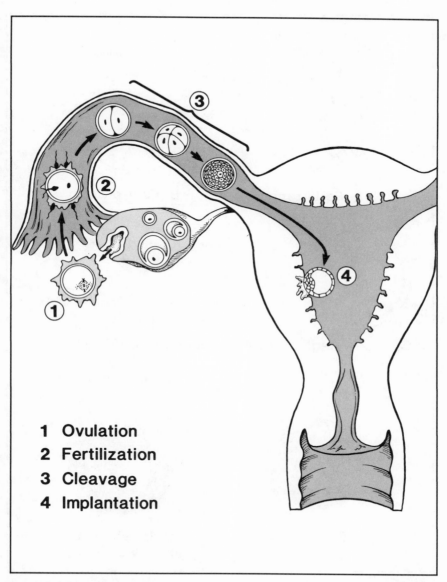

1 Ovulation
2 Fertilization
3 Cleavage
4 Implantation

Events Leading to Implantation   **Figure 3**
The egg, fertilized in the upper reaches of the fallopian tube, divides (cleaves) numerous times before implanting in the uterus.

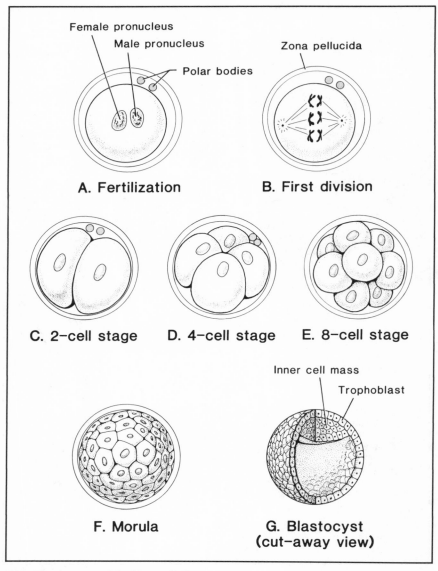

Early Development of the Human Embryo   **Figure 4**

A series of cleavage divisions leads to a 6-day embryo, the blastocyst, *which resembles a hollow sphere. The aggregation of cells at one pole, called the* inner cell mass, *is destined to form the fetus itself. The outer rim of cells, the* trophoblast, *will ultimately contribute to the formation of the placenta.*

In the initial trials at establishing pregnancy, Edwards and Steptoe employed ovulation-inducing drugs to improve the chances of recovering eggs from the ovary. However, they became convinced that the use of such fertility drugs so depressed the hormonal state of the woman as to interfere with the proper implantation of the embryo in the uterus. Indeed, in the absence of a suitable hormonal environment to prepare the uterus, the embryo may lodge in ectopic sites such as the fallopian tubes. Stated another way, tubal pregnancies tend to be fostered when inappropriate hormonal conditions make the uterus unreceptive. In the late 1970s, Edwards and Steptoe discontinued the use of fertility drugs and relied almost exclusively on the spontaneous hormonal cycle of the woman.[10] They scheduled the laparoscopic aspiration at twenty-four to twenty-eight hours after the body's natural surge of the particular hormone (luteinizing hormone) that normally triggers ovulation. The most notable outcome of depending on the natural ovulatory cycle of the woman was Mrs. Brown's successful pregnancy.

When it was established that pregnancy had occurred, Mrs. Brown was sent home and encouraged to live a normal but restful life. She returned to Oldham Hospital for a series of tests throughout the pregnancy, staying in the hospital for two or three days on each occasion. She was examined periodically by ultrasonic scan; amniocentesis under ultrasound scrutiny was performed at approximately sixteen weeks of gestation. The amniotic cells were harvested for chromosomal analysis.[11] As reported by Steptoe and

---

[10]A discouraging aspect of placing one's trust in the spontaneous ovulatory cycle with the release of only a single egg is the low pregnancy rate of about ten percent. When more than one ovarian egg is stimulated to mature by the use of fertility drugs (clomiphene citrate and human menopausal gonadotropin), the success rate is improved appreciably to be about 20 percent. The greater pregnancy rate is to be weighed against the potential adverse outcome of tubal ectopic pregnancy. The occurrence of ectopic pregnancies after *in vitro* fertilization is being increasingly recognized in several centers. See D. M. Bearman, P. A. Vieta, Richard D. Snipes, R. P. Gobien, et al., "Heterotopic Pregnancy After *in Vitro* Fertilization and Embryo Transfer," *Fertility and Sterility* 45 (1986): 719-21.

[11]The technique of amniocentesis has become an important tool in the prenatal detection of certain hereditary disorders. The technique consists of inserting a hypodermic needle into the uterus of the expectant mother, and withdrawing a small sample of amniotic fluid. The cells of the amniotic fluid are then examined both biochemically and chromosomally. Analysis of the chromosome complement permits the identification of the sex of the fetus. Among the abnormalities detectable by amniocentesis are Down syndrome, neural tube defects, enzyme deficiencies (as in Tay-Sachs disease and Lesch-Nyhan syndrome), and hemoglobinopathies (sickle cell anemia and thalassemia).

Edwards, the analyses "revealed normal α-fetoprotein levels, with no chromosome abnormalities in 46 XX fetus."[12] That the analysis revealed a normal fetus came as a great relief to the Browns. The XX chromosomal constitution indicated that the fetus was a female. Although the sex of the baby was determined in advance from the chromosomal tests, Mrs. Brown did not want to be informed because, in her words, she "did not want to be cheated of the final thrill."

The birth of Louise Brown immediately brought into focus a number of sensitive ethical issues.[13] For some philosophers and theologians, *in vitro* fertilization represents another dehumanizing step toward subverting reverence for life.[14] Paul Ramsey of Princeton University, a conservative Protestant theologian, contends that *in vitro* fertilization is inherently an immoral form of procreation.[15] The procedure is "unnatural" and erodes the union of personal love with procreation. He feels that it is not a proper goal of medicine to enable women to become pregnant artificially, nor to interfere with natural fecundity. Ramsey is unwavering in the belief that for human reproduction to be moral, the act must be coital or natural. Adherents of this claim might even suggest that other artificial technologies undermine both the individual and the family. Indeed, extreme absolutists

---

[12]The birth of Louise Joy Brown was first reported in a very brief communication on 12 August 1978 by P. C. Steptoe and R. G. Edwards (*Lancet* 2 [1971]: 366).

[13]For a thorough survey of the literature of ethical issues concerned with new reproductive technologies, see Leroy Walters, "Human *in Vitro* Fertilization: A Review of the Ethical Literature," *The Hastings Center Report* 9: (1979) 23-43.

[14]The Vatican reiterates the Church's long-standing position that interference with nature in any form is not acceptable. The Papacy has pronounced authoritatively against artificial insemination, even with the husband as a donor. Jewish religious authorities, on the whole, respond favorably to *in vitro* fertilization, since a woman, clearly designated as barren, can now bear children. The favorable attitude of rabbinical authorities is based on the biblical commandment: "Be fertile and multiply; fill the earth and multiply it" (Genesis 1:28). On the other hand, there is the possibility of egg (and sperm) wastage in the procedures, which according to Jewish religion, is forbidden on the basis of the biblical injunction against "spilling of the seed needlessly." See J. G. Schenker, "Jewish and Moslem Aspects of *in Vitro* Fertilization and Embryo Transfer," *Annals of the New York Academy of Sciences* 442 (1985): 601-607.

[15]P. Ramsey, "Shall We 'Reproduce'? The Medical Ethics of *in Vitro* Fertilization," *Journal of the American Medical Association* 220 (1972): 1346-50; "Shall We 'Reproduce'? II. Rejoinders and Future Forecast," *Journal of the American Medical Association* 220 (1972): 1480-85.

would condemn anything that is artificial, including vaccination against infectious disease, life-saving kidney transplants, the administration of drugs, the bottle feeding of infants, and a host of other medical technologies. If we were to reject medical advances on the premise that they were unnatural, then we would have to renounce the whole essence of the medical enterprise, which exists to correct the deficiencies of nature.

An open-minded outlook is implicit in the writings of Joseph Fletcher, a liberal Protestant ethicist at the University of Virginia Medical School.[16] Fletcher is less concerned with prescribed rules and addresses in concrete terms the moral quandaries that actually confront a person in everyday life. Rightness or wrongness are judged according to results, not according to absolute prohibition. Fletcher strongly defends the new technology and asserts that the benefits of the procedure clearly outweigh the perceived or actual detriments. He dismisses abstract concepts and directs his attention to actual human needs and human desires. The desire to have children justifies a woman's desire to undertake *in vitro* fertilization.

Medicine tends to be guided by the utilitarian principle of beneficence. That is to say, the course of action that produces the most beneficial effects and the least harmful effects is held to be the best action to take. Accordingly, the conduct of medicine is measured in terms of the good produced for the patient. The ability to have a child satisfies one of the most profound human needs, and the expectation is that physicians would employ the most advanced medical techniques to help couples fulfill themselves as parents. It would be ideal if the medical profession could effortlessly remedy all tubal disabilities, but a cure is usually very difficult or impossible. Much of medical therapy is directed towards alleviating a deficiency rather than producing a cure. Nevertheless, some professional scientists have advocated that the infertile woman should forsake child-producing therapy to await a cure for her tubal problem. In particular, Leon Kass of the National Institutes of Health maintains that the desire to have a child, although a worthy craving, does not legitimize medical intervention.[17] He chastises the medical profession for treating a desire rather than the dis-

---

[16]J. Fletcher, "*In Vitro* Fertilization of Human Ova and Blastocyst Transfer: An Invitational Symposium," *Journal of Reproductive Medicine* 11 (1972): 198.

[17]L. R. Kass, "Making Babies—the New Biology and the 'Old' Morality," *Public Interest* 26 (1972): 32-33; "Babies by Means of *in Vitro* Fertilization: Unethical experiments on the unborn," *New England Journal of Medicine* 285 (1971): 1176-77.

ease. Instead of repairing the blocked fallopian tube, the physician is gratifying the longing of the woman to have a child. In an argument that is
scarcely credible to most medical practitioners, Kass expects the physician
to treat the cause of the problem (the blocked tube) but not the effect (her
childlessness).

Aspiring parents have sought the technique of *in vitro* fertilization for
a variety of medical reasons. The technique provides a means of overcoming a form of female infertility in which the fallopian tubes are blocked,
scarred, or missing. Malfunctioning tubes account for approximately twenty
percent of the cases of infertility. Women with markedly scarred tubes
cannot be treated with conventional surgical procedures. The technique of
in vitro fertilization can also be helpful to those women who fail to conceive because the chemical fluids in the cervical canal have deleterious effects on the sperm. Additionally, some men suffer from low sperm counts;
this condition, known as oligospermia, is as refractory to medical treatment as extensive tubal damage. Such oligospermic men can benefit from
in vitro fertilization because fewer sperm cells are required compared with
the massive numbers needed naturally. In sharp contrast to the five million
normally required, as few as 50,000 viable sperm can serve the purpose *in
vitro*. In essence, an appreciable number of hopeful parents have no alternative chance of conception—all other methods having failed.

The collaborative work of Steptoe and Edwards at Oldham hospital
stopped, at least temporarily, shortly after the birth of Louise Brown. Patrick Steptoe had reached the age of retirement from the National Health
Service, and increasing demands had been placed on Robert Edwards at
Cambridge University. No longer was it feasible to carry out the long-dis-
tance cooperation of former years. It took a span of two years for the two
investigators to re-establish a new clinic in Bourn Hall, near Cambridge.
Patients came to Bourn from all over the world. In the relatively short period between October 1980, when the Bourn Clinic opened its doors, to
May 1984, the clinic recorded 439 pregnancies, of which 131 were ongoing. Two hundred fifteen children have been born since the inception of
the clinic, including eighteen sets of twins and one set of triplets. There
have been no major congenital malformations in the infants. Among the
mothers of this new clinic was Lesley Brown, who delivered her second
child, Natalie Jane, conceived by the *in vitro* fertilization technique, on 15
June 1982.

Numerous *in vitro* fertilization clinics have since emerged in other parts
of the world. In 1979, several investigators from two universities in Mel-

bourne, Australia—Monash University and the University of Melbourne—collaborated to duplicate the success of Edwards and Steptoe.[18] The two Melbourne teams now work independently in their respective universities.[19] It was at Melbourne that the first human infant was born who had grown from an embryo that had been frozen and then thawed. In 1980 the technology was introduced in the United States by Drs. Howard and Georgeanna Jones at Eastern Virginia Medical School in Norfolk.[20] This original program still reigns as one of the most highly successful American programs. The Norfolk team pioneered the use of human menopausal gonadotropin (hMG) in order to enhance the chance of pregnancy by having available multiple eggs for fertilization and transfer. There are currently in excess of 100 private facilities in the United States, with many more on the horizon.

In vitro fertilization is no longer only of academic interest, to be taken lightly. The procedure has gone beyond the research stage and can now be considered as an established form of treatment for infertility. Presently, *in vitro* fertilization clinics have been established in about 28 countries.[21] It is not inconceivable that an *in vitro* fertilization program will, in the not too distant future, be part of the standard gynecologic services offered at major medical centers.[22] Parenthood, even when it originates in the laboratory, is still an exalted event.

---

[18]A. Lopata, I. W. H. Johnston, I. J. Hoult, and A. I. Speirs, "Pregnancy Following Intrauterine Implantation of an Embryo Obtained by *in Vitro* Fertilization of a Preovulatory Egg," *Fertility and Sterility* 33 (1980): 117-20.

[19]I. Johnson, A. Lopata, A. I. Speirs, A. J. Hoult, G. Kellow and Y. DuPlessis, "*In Vitro* Fertilization: The Challenge of the Eighties," *Fertility and Sterility* 36 (1981): 691-706; A. O. Trounson, J. F. Leeton, C. Wood, J. Wood, "Pregnancies in Humans by Fertilization *in Vitro* and Embryo Transfer in the Controlled Ovulatory Cycle," *Science* 212 (1981): 681-82.

[20]H. W. Jones, A. A. Acosta, M. C. Andrews, J. E. Garcia, et al., "Three Years of *in Vitro* Fertilization at Norfolk," *Fertility and Sterility* 42 (1984): 826-34.

[21]These countries include Argentina, Australia, Austria, Belgium, Canada, Chile, Columbia, England, Finland, France, India, Indonesia, Israel, Italy, Japan, Mexico, Netherlands, People's Republic of China, Peru, Singapore, South Africa, Spain, Sweden, Switzerland, Taiwan, Thailand, United States, and West Germany.

[22]A worldwide survey conducted by the Finnish physician Markku Seppälä indicated that between 1978 and 31 January 1984, 590 births have resulted from 517 *in vitro* pregnancies and 570 clinical pregnancies were still ongoing. Most of the pregnancies have resulted in single births, but there have been fifty-six sets of twins, seven sets of triplets, and two sets of quadruplets. See M. Seppälä, "The World Collaborative Report on *in Vitro* Fertilization and Embryo Replacement: Current State of the Art in January 1984," *Annals of the New York Academy of Sciences* 442 (1985): 558-68.

Chapter 2

America's Experience

America was late in establishing *in vitro* fertilization clinics. In the 1970s, critics questioned the propriety of manipulating the human embryo without knowledge of the hidden risks. Anxieties mounted that the clinical use of *in vitro* fertilization was premature and hazardous. In 1975, almost all government-sponsored research with human eggs came to an abrupt halt in the United States. Under 1975 federal order, the Department of Health, Education, and Welfare (HEW) was barred from funding any research project involving *in vitro* fertilization unless the proposed program was first approved by a national Ethics Advisory Board appointed by the HEW secretary. No such advisory board was appointed until the birth of Britain's first test-tube baby.

In July 1978, spurred by the wave of public interest in the birth of baby Brown, the then HEW Secretary, Joseph A. Califano, called for national hearings on whether the United States should finance research that could lead to a similar birth in the United States.[1] The composition of HEW's

---

[1] With the announcement of the birth of Louise Brown in England, the American news media inquired at government agencies about comparable research endeavors by American scientists. In 1978, the National Institutes of Health had on record only one pending research proposal, entitled "Cytogenetics of Human Preimplantation Embryos," which had been submitted by Dr. Pierre Soupart, Professor of Obstetrics and Gynecology at Vanderbilt University Medical Center, Nashville, Tennessee. Dr. Soupart died in 1981 before ever receiving a final decision regarding federal support of his research proposal that languished in the hands of the Secretary of HEW.

thirteen-member Ethics Advisory Board was mixed: lawyers, obstetricians, surgeons, geneticists, medical ethicists, and businessmen.[2] Mr. Califano stated that research in the field of reproductive science not only would enable many barren women to bear children, but might produce knowledge that could help physicians alleviate genetic diseases. He hastened to add, however, that the novel procedures raise serious ethical questions, including the possibility of unscrupulous experiments on human embryos. The Ethics Advisory Board held hearings in many cities at which numerous speakers testified, and reviewed diligently well over two thousand letters from public interest groups and private individuals. Infertile couples responded overwhelmingly in favor of risking the new reproductive technologies in order to have their own biological offspring.

A comprehensive two-volume document was prepared by the Ethics Advisory Board in 1979.[3] The report stated unequivocally that research on human *in vitro* fertilization is acceptable from an ethical standpoint provided that strict procedures are observed. However, to this day, with each change of administration, the extant Secretary of HEW (now Health and Human Services, or HHS) has ignored the Board's recommendation. The Ethics Advisory Board has ceased to exist, and no federal grants have yet been approved to support clinical human trials on *in vitro* fertilization.

The report of the HEW Ethics Advisory Board stressed the desirability of additional research in order to assess the risks to both mother and offspring. Assurance of the normalcy of the *in vitro* fertilized egg was con-

---

[2]The members of the Ethics Advisory Board of the Department of Health, Education, and Welfare were as follows: James C. Gaither, San Francisco laywer, chairman; David A. Hamburg, president, Institute of Medicine of the National Academy of Sciences, vice-chairman; Sissela Bok, lecturer in Medical Ethics, Harvard University; Jack T. Conway, senior vice-president, United Way of America; Henry W. Foster, professor and chairman, Obstetrics and Gynecology Department, Meharry Medical College; Donald A. Henderson, dean, School of Hygiene and Public Health, Johns Hopkins University; Maurice Lazarus, executive, Federated Department Stores, Inc., Boston; Richard A. McCormick, professor of Christian Ethics, Kennedy Institute for the Study of Reproduction and Bioethics, Georgetown University; Robert F. Murray, chief, Medical Genetics Division, Howard University College of Medicine; Mitchell W. Spellman, dean for Medical Services, Harvard University Medical School; Daniel C. Tosteson, dean, Harvard University Medical School; Agnes N. Williams, laywer, Potomac, Maryland; and Eugene M. Zweiback, surgeon, Omaha, Nebraska.

[3]Ethics Advisory Board. HEW support of research involving human *in vitro* fertilization and embryo transfer. Two volumes: *Report* and *Conclusions,* and an appendix (Washington DC: Department of Health, Education, and Welfare, 4 May 1979).

sidered one of the more critical problems. Few investigators have had the opportunity to observe the development of human embryos. The Ethics Advisory Board proposed a systematic exploration of the chromosomal makeup of human embryos produced in culture to determine whether or not the chromosomal complements are markedly altered from those of embryos produced by the normal reproductive process. But, the only way to make such an assessment is to undertake comprehensive research, which HEW has yet to sanction. Providentially, although the experience to date is inconclusive, the existing findings indicate that the technique of *in vitro* fertilization neither fosters aberrant chromosomal changes nor favors the survival of embryos that do have chromosomal abnormalities. In essence, the knowable risks to the baby are equivalent to the risks normally undertaken in a natural pregnancy.[4]

The Federal moratorium on human *in vitro* fertilization research has not impeded the clinical application of the technique in the United States. The American clinical centers that have been established are all privately funded, with patient fees contributing to the conduct of research. The failure of the Federal government to oversee or monitor the technology may have actually intensified the incentive of the private sector to act. Ironically, then, *in vitro* fertilization in the United States has passed through the early phases of technological development to clinical application without any government intrusion. The procedure also has become part of clinical practice without pervasive public scrutiny.[5] Well over 100 *in vitro* centers presently exist in the United States (figure 5).

---

[4]The Ethics Advisory Board acknowledged concern that technological intervention might encourage unwholesome genetic manipulation of the human embryo. However, the Board recognized that there is an opportunity for abuse in the application of any novel technology, and that this concern in itself could not justify the prohibition of research on *in vitro* fertilization in humans.

[5]In contrast to the United States, the establishment of *in vitro* centers in Britain and Australia has been accompanied by appreciable public discussion. The most recent committee of citizens in England to evaluate the social, ethical, and legal issues was chaired by Dame Mary Warnock, Mistress of Girton College in Cambridge (*Report of the Committee of Inquiry into Human Fertilization and Embryology,* Department of Health and Social Security, Her Majesty's Stationery Office, London, 1984). An equally comprehensive report by a public group in Australia was published in 1982 (Committee to Consider the Social, Ethical, and Legal Issues Arising from *In Vitro* Fertilization, *Interim Report to the Attorney General,* State of Victoria, Australia, September, 1982).

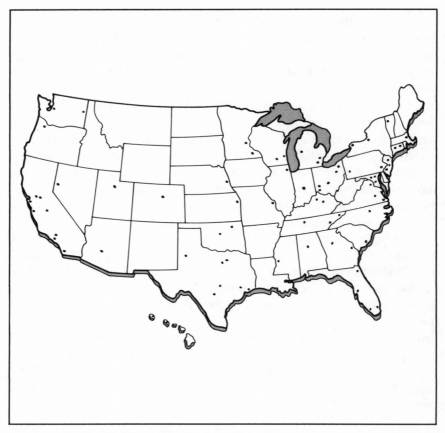

Location of *in Vitro* Fertilization Clinics in the United States   **Figure 5**

Birmingham AL, Phoenix AZ, Berkeley CA, Northridge CA, Sacramento CA, San Fran-cisco CA, Walnut Creek CA, Whittier CA, Fresno CA, La Jolla CA, Los Angeles CA, Den-ver CO, Farmington CT, Hartford CT, New Haven CT, Washington DC, Jacksonville FL, Miami FL, Naples FL, Tampa FL, Atlanta GA, Augusta GA, Honolulu HI, Lihue HI, Chi-cago IL, Indianapolis IN, Kansas City KS, Lexington KY, Louisville KY, New Orleans LA, Baltimore MD, Bethesda MD, Boston MA, Newton MA, Ann Arbor MI, Grand Rapids MI, Detroit MI, Royal Oak MI, Minneapolis MN, Rochester MN, Jackson MS, St. Louis MO, Omaha NE, Reno NV, Stratford NJ, Newark NJ, New Brunswick NJ, Buffalo NY, Dobbs Ferry NY, New York NY, Manhasset NY, Port Chester NY, Rochester NY, Chapel Hill NC, Durham NC, Akron OH, Cincinnati OH, Cleveland OH, Columbus OH, Dayton OH, Oklahoma City OK, Tulsa OK, Portland OR, Elkins Park PA, Philadelphia PA, Pittsburgh PA, Charleston SC, Johnson City TN, Knoxville TN, Nashville TN, Austin TX, Carrollton TX, Dallas TX, Fort Worth TX, Galveston TX, Houston TX, Lubbock TX, San Antonio TX, Salt Lake City UT, Burlington VT, Fairfax VA, Norfolk VA, Richmond VA, Seattle WA, Spokane WA, Madison WI, Milwaukee WI, Waukesha WI.

America's first test-tube baby was born in late 1981. At 7:46 a.m. on 28 December 1981, in Norfolk, Virginia, a normal five-pound, twelve-ounce Elizabeth Jane Carr was delivered by caesarean section to Judith Carr, a twenty-eight-year-old Westminster, Massachusetts, schoolteacher. The conception and birth were supervised by Dr. Howard Jones, a gynecological surgeon, and his wife, Dr. Georgeanna Jones, a reproductive endocrinologist, at Norfolk General Hospital, which is affiliated with the Eastern Virginia Medical School. Coincidentally, Elizabeth Carr's birth weight was precisely the same as Louise Brown's had been at birth.

Drs. Howard and Georgeanna Jones had each retired earlier as professors of gynecology and obstetrics from the Johns Hopkins University, where they had earned an international reputation over a thirty-five-year period for their work on human infertility. They arrived in Norfolk for a quiet life of semi-retirement on the very day that Louise Brown was born in Britain. When the local press asked them in an interview whether an *in vitro clinic* could be established in Norfolk, the Joneses responded in the affirmative. Although the positive nod was not meant to be a firm declaration of intent, a clinic was launched three years later with private donations. One large contribution came from a grateful woman who, earlier in her life, had achieved pregnancy after medical treatments by Georgeanna Jones.

The Joneses weathered a barrage of criticism from those who wished to prevent the establishment of the *in vitro* fertilization clinic at Norfolk. The Joneses survived the stormy public hearings and opened their clinic on 1 March 1980. They also survived a very sobering initiation period. They went through an initial 45 laparoscopies before achieving their first successful pregnancy. Today, their success rate is one pregnancy for every four embryos transferred.[6] Their success reflects, among other things, the controlled use of ovulation-inducing hormones to enhance the chances of obtaining fertilizable eggs from the ovary.

There is no shortage of women opting for the procedure. Only married couples are allowed to participate in the program at Norfolk, so that the resulting babies are the products of their own parents.[7] Several couples have

---

[6]Jones, H. W., et al., "Three Years of *in Vitro* Fertilization in Norfolk," *Fertility and Sterility* 42 (1984): 826-34.

[7]Although many clinics have adopted the policy that only married couples can avail themselves of *in vitro* fertilization, such a limitation might be an unconstitutional depri-

adopted children, but the compelling urge is for offspring that are biologically their own. The women jokingly refer to themselves as "mother hens," "incubators," and "good eggs." Each month-long session at Norfolk costs a couple about $5,500. The demand is substantial; there are three to four thousand women waiting to get on the six-month list. This represents more than a ten-year backlog, inasmuch as the clinic can handle only 270 patients a year. The surfeit of patients is an expression of the overwhelming desire of infertile couples to have children at any cost.[8]

It takes a well-structured, experienced team to run a demanding and exacting *in vitro* fertilization program. In 1984, the American Fertility Society arranged for a committee, headed by Dr. Howard Jones, to establish minimal standards for initiating a clinical program. The standards ensure that quality control is maintained at every step in the procedure and at all times.[9] In 1986, the American Fertility Society addressed the ethical issues involved in the reproductive technologies.[10] The impressive deliberations of the American Fertility Society are intended to take the place of federal regulations, which presently do not exist. The absence of federal regula-

---

vation of equal protection to unmarried infertile couples. Since there is no medical basis for differentiating between married infertile persons and unmarried infertile persons, the latter individuals could argue that such a limitation abridges their right of procreation. See M. M. Quigley and L. B. Andrews, "Human *in Vitro* Fertilization and the Law," *Fertility and Sterility* 42 (1984): 348-55.

[8]There are a number of anecdotal stories that dispel the oft-stated assertion of conservative moral theologians that *in vitro* fertilization represents a degradation of parenthood. When one woman at Norfolk was informed of her pregnant state, she remarked that it was the first time she felt a strong bond of love between her and her husband. Another proud mother kept a diary of her several weeks at Norfolk to show her child the extent of her determination and longing. More than one couple requested the plastic culture dishes in which fertilization occurred, so that their children would know exactly where they were conceived. Evidently, an *in vitro* baby is unique and special to a previously infertile couple.

[9]A team approach is essential for an *in vitro* fertilization program to function efficiently and consistently on a daily basis. There should be personnel with expertise in gynecology, laparoscopy, andrology (male reproduction), tissue culture methodology, reproductive biology (fertilization and early embryonic development), and reproductive endocrinology (hormones). Services and hospital facilities should be available for ultrasonography, hormonal assays, anesthesia, follicular aspiration, and embryo transfer. An operating theatre with its own staff and an adjacent laboratory for fertilization and culture are imperative. See American Fertility Society, "Minimal Standards for Programs of *in Vitro* Fertilization," *Fertility and Sterility* 41 (1984): 13-14.

[10]The Ethics Committee of the American Fertility Society, "Ethical Considerations of the New Reproductive Technologies," *Fertility and Sterility* 46, Supplement 1 (1986): 1-94.

tions, however, does not preempt state regulations. Subject to federal constitutional constraints, states do have the freedom to regulate or monitor the new reproductive capabilities. With the exception of a most unusual statute in Illinois, no state has explicitly regulated *in vitro* fertilization.[11] There are, however, existing laws in many states that might be interpreted as precluding the practice of *in vitro* fertilization. Twenty-five states have statutes on the books that prohibit experimentation on fetuses or abortuses. Thus, depending on whether the word "fetus" is explicitly defined to include the embryo, the manipulation of the embryo in the culture dish or its transfer to the mother could be construed as experimentation on a fetus. However, if the fetal laws of the states are ever viewed as sufficiently broad to place restraints on the ability of an infertile woman to avail herself of *in vitro* fertilization, it is likely that the state laws would be challenged as infringing on the woman's constitutional right to make procreative decisions.[12]

One of the largest private clinics in the United States is located in Port Chester, New York, operated by a corporation called IVF Australia. The clinic claims that it can take care of one thousand women a year, at least twice the capabilities of the Norfolk clinic. The Port Chester clinic was established by Vicki Baldwin, an American who several years ago had availed herself of the *in vitro* program at Monash University in Melbourne, Australia. After having had two children as a result of the treatment, Baldwin negotiated a contract with Monash University that gives her corporation in the United States exclusive rights to the commercial application of the procedures used by the Monash University *in vitro* team.

Based on the capabilities of the Monash group, the Port Chester Clinic offers a procedure that has raised concern even among American physicians. The unorthodox procedure involves the freezing of embryos, storing them for weeks or months, and then thawing them out for transfer into the woman's womb. The "freeze-thaw" technique is acceptable in Aus-

---

[11]The Illinois law specifically makes a physician who fertilizes a woman's egg outside her body criminally liable if the physician endangers the life or health of the embryo. Thus, broad sanctions are imposed on Illinois physicians, but the parameters of these sanctions are not clearly explained.

[12]Various legal questions involving *in vitro* fertilization and fetal research are discussed lucidly by an attorney, Lori B. Andrews, in *New Conceptions: A Consumer's Guide to the Newest Infertility Treatments Including In Vitro Fertilizations, Artificial Insemination, and Surrogate Motherhood* (New York: Ballantine Books, 1985).

tralia, where at least a dozen healthy babies have been produced from previously frozen embryos. The first of such births occurred in Melbourne in the spring of 1984 (see chapter 6).

The Port Chester Clinic has lost out in its quest to have the nation's first birth using the "freeze-thaw" procedure. This singular distinction, considered dubious by some, belongs to a clinic associated with the University of Southern California School of Medicine. The clinic is housed at the Hospital of the Good Samaritan, under the direction of Dr. Richard Marrs. On Wednesday, 4 June 1986, a nine-pound, ten-ounce boy was delivered to a grateful couple, who earlier had expressed reservation that their frozen embryo, after thawing, would develop normally.[13]

At present, there is no ethical or legal framework in the United States to regulate the "freeze-thaw" procedure.[14] Some authors have argued for increasing involvement of the Federal government in decisions concerning the newer reproductive capabilities. There are, however, a number of compelling arguments against establishing federal regulations. The most cogent reason is to guard against unwarranted governmental intrusion into matters so fundamentally affecting a person as the decision to bear a child, even if it entails sophisticated medical technology.[15]

------

[13]The Associated Press, "First in U.S.: Healthy Boy is Born After Frozen Embryo Implantation," *The Atlanta Journal,* 5 June 1986.

[14]C. Grobstein, M. Flower, and J. Mendeloff, "Frozen Embryos: Policy Issues," *New England Journal of Medicine* 312 (1985): 1484-1588.

[15]Like so many other occasions when the Federal government attempts to legislate morality, more distress is created than is relieved. This is vividly demonstrated by the unwarranted and unreasonable federal intrusion on the practice of withholding medical treatment from handicapped infants. On 18 May 1982, the U.S. Department of Health and Human Services issued a notice informing hospitals that they could lose federal assistance if medical or surgical treatment was withheld from a handicapped infant. On June 9, 1986, the Supreme Court invalidated the HHS regulation that was designed to require life-prolonging treatment for handicapped newborn infants. The opinion of the Supreme Court was that there was no basis for an insensitive Federal regulation that effectively prevents parents from having the determining influence, if not final say, on delicate decisions concerning their offspring.

Chapter 3

State of the Arts

Infertility is a disheartening state that touches the lives of one of eight women of childbearing age. In the United States alone, four million couples have experienced the anxiety of trying unsuccessfully for several years to conceive. Many couples encounter infertility early in their married lives and find it difficult to cope with this life crisis. A profound sense of helplessness and hopelessness accompanies the reality of barrenness. An unspoken fear of each spouse is the loss of a once-strong marital relationship. As society places a premium on parenthood, infertile couples often feel that their self-worth is lessened by their inability to produce children.[1] For many couples, *in vitro* fertilization represents the end of a long, agonizing search to overcome their childlessness.

Most couples enrolled in an *in vitro* fertilization program have a lengthy history of infertility, some extending as long as fifteen years. Most have availed themselves of the usual fertility treatments, and all are consumed by the drive to achieve their goal to conceive. Their aspirations remain high, even when confronted with the statistical realities of failure of the *in vitro*

---

[1] That infertility is an insult to a person's self-esteem is aptly described in the following quotation: "My infertility is a blow to my self-esteem, a violation of my privacy, an assault on my sexuality, a final exam on my ability to cope, an affront to my sense of justice, a painful reminder that nothing can be taken for granted. My infertility is a break in the continuity of life. It is above all, a wound—to my body, to my psyche, to my soul." (M. A. Jorgenson, "On Healing," *Resolve Newsletter* [December, 1981]: 1).

program. The majority of the patients who enter the program are women with tubal problems. Other participants are oligospermic males and infertile women with tubal complications resulting from endometriosis. Still others are ostensibly normal couples who are infertile for reasons that escape our current medical understanding. Some men, for example, have normal sperm counts and motility, but their sperm inexplicably lack the ability to penetrate the outer thick coating of the egg. Women over forty are rarely encouraged to participate because the risk factors are too great and the chances of success are slim. Aside from a less supportive womb for embryo implantation, older women experience an increased incidence of chromosomally abnormal conceptuses, the most notable being Down syndrome.[2]

Women are endowed with far more eggs than they will ever need during their child-bearing years. The paired, compact ovaries at birth harbor as many as two million potential eggs. Starting at puberty (ages eleven to fourteen), eggs are released, usually one at a time each month, about midway of the menstrual cycle (figure 6). Scarcely any eggs are present by the time the woman reaches menopause (ages forty-five to fifty). All the potential eggs for the human female are found in her ovaries when she is born; there is not a continual renewal of eggs throughout the reproductive years.

Figure 7 illustrates the development of an egg in the ovary. At an early stage, the potential egg is surrounded by a single layer of nourishing cells, called follicle cells.[3] The combination of egg and follicle cells is called a

---

[2]The effects of maternal age on fecundity and fertility are reviewed by R. G. Gosden in "Maternal Age: A Major Factor Affecting Prospects and Outcome of Pregnancy," *Annals of the New York Academy of Sciences* 442 (1985): 45-57.

[3]The "egg" in the developing follicle is technically a *primary oocyte*. Fertilization cannot take place unless the primary oocyte undergoes maturational changes, which involve two successive cell divisions called *meiotic divisions*. The primary oocyte in the ovary remains arrested in the prophase of the first meiotic division until the onset of sexual maturity. Under the influence of appropriate hormones, the primary oocyte resumes and completes the first meiotic division to become a *secondary oocyte*. At this point, the second meiotic division ensues. When released from the surface of the ovary during ovulation, the secondary oocyte is seen to be arrested in the metaphase of the second meiotic division. The stimulus for the resumption of the second meiotic division is normally the penetration of the secondary oocyte by the sperm cell. The egg completes the second meiotic division by releasing a set of chromosomes in a polar body and retaining a haploid set of twenty-three chromosomes, comparable to the haploid male set of twenty-three chromosomes contributed by the sperm.

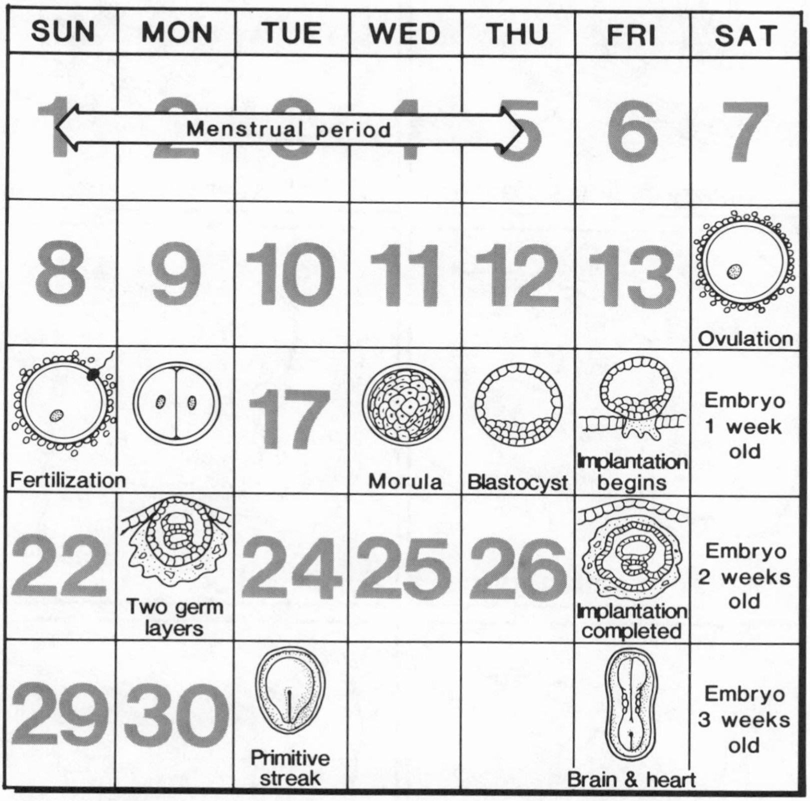

SUN	MON	TUE	WED	THU	FRI	SAT
1	2	3	4	5	6	7
(Menstrual period)						
8	9	10	11	12	13	Ovulation
Fertilization		17	Morula	Blastocyst	Implantation begins	Embryo 1 week old
22	Two germ layers	24	25	26	Implantation completed	Embryo 2 weeks old
29	30	Primitive streak			Brain & heart	Embryo 3 weeks old

Main Events during Early Pregnancy

Figure 6

Given that the menstrual period is the first five days, ovulation typically occurs on the fourteenth day and implantation (assuming fertilization) takes place on the twentieth day. The three-week-old embryo has the rudiments of brain and heart.

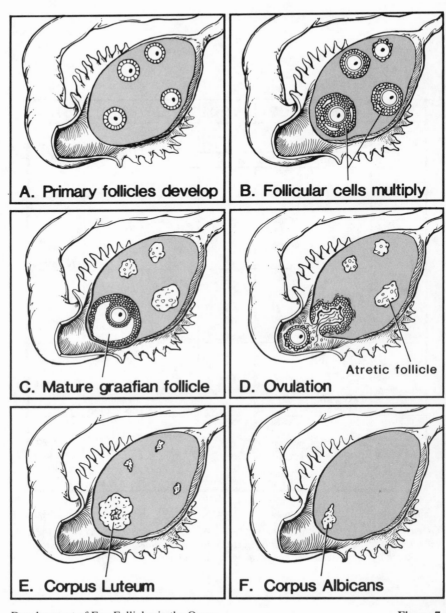

Development of Egg Follicles in the Ovary   **Figure 7**
Of the four immature (primary) follicles, one grows into a mature (Graafian) follicle and three others disintegrate (undergo atresia). After ovulation, the mature follicle persists as the corpus luteum (if pregnancy occurs) or becomes white scar tissue, the corpus albicans (if the pregnancy does not take place).

primary follicle. As the egg enlarges (matures), the follicle cells multiply to form several layers and the egg becomes protected in a fluid-filled cavity. The fully developed follicle, or *Graafian follicle,* appears as a very thin and translucent bulge at the surface of the ovary. The rounded and turgid follicle resembles a blister and eventually ruptures. The liberation of the egg from the ruptured follicle constitutes *ovulation.*

Normally, each month, several primary follicles begin to enlarge simultaneously, but usually only one reaches maturity and ruptures to release an egg. The spurious development and degeneration of a follicle is called *atresia.*[4] Occasionally, however, two or more follicles mature, and more than one egg is released. Successful fertilization of the multiple eggs may lead to multiple births; in such an event, the sibling offspring are fraternal (nonidentical). The changes associated with the development of a primary follicle into a mature Graafian follicle are brought about by specific hormones (gonadotropins) secreted by the pituitary gland. These pituitary gonadotropins or their synthetic analogs have been used therapeutically in women with hormonal dysfunctions. Ovulation can be successfully induced or stimulated by the administration of the pituitary gonadotropins.

Our understanding of the action of the gonadotropins has been used in the *in vitro* fertilization procedure to recover the egg at a time when the follicles are ripe but as yet unruptured. Rather than rely uncertainly on the unpredictable natural hormonal cycle of the woman, investigators have found that the onset of ovulation can be accurately timed by the administration of pituitary gonadotropins or their counterparts. The ovulation-inducing agents actually cause several follicles to mature simultaneously. The recovery of larger numbers of fertilizable eggs at the time of laparoscopy is translated into higher pregnancy rates.[5]

---

[4]Once a follicle emerges from the resting pool, it must continue to mature or succumb to atresia. Apparently the follicle destined for ovulation secretes a substance that inhibits the development of other potentially competing follicles. G. D. Hodgen, "The dominant ovarian follicle," *Fertility and Sterility* 38 (1982): 281-301.

[5]Several scientific treatises are now available that provide extensive information on varied aspects of *in vitro* fertilization as related to individual clinics in different countries. See R. G. Edwards and J. M. Purdy, eds., *Human Conception in Vitro* (London: Academic Press, 1982); W. A. W. Walters and P. Singer, eds., *Test-Tube Babies* (New York: Oxford University Press, 1982); H. M. Beier and H. R. Lindner, eds., *Fertilization of the Human Egg in Vitro* (New York: Springer-Verlag, 1983); C. Wood and A. Trounson, eds. *Clinical In*

Multiple follicle stimulation is generally achieved through the use of Clomid (clomiphene citrate) in combination with human menopausal gonadotropin (hMG), or hMG alone. Clomid activates the hormonal controlling center in the brain and hMG encourages the follicles to mature.[6] Figure 8 shows a sample cycle, which begins with day one of the menstrual cycle (first day of menses). From day three to day eight of the cycle, the woman takes a prescribed dose of Clomid orally every morning. Starting on day eight and for several days thereafter, one or more ampules of hMG are injected in the woman intramuscularly, the injection procedure typically being performed by the husband.

The growth of the follicle is assessed in two ways: the ovary is examined regularly by ultrasound scan and the level of estrogen (estradiol) circulating in the blood is measured routinely.[7] When the estrogen levels and ultrasound images indicate that ovulation is imminent, the women receives a single dose of human chorionic gonadotropin (hCG), which is remarkably similar to luteinizing hormone (LH). Like LH, the hCG triggers, within thirty-six hours, the release of the egg from the bulging Graafian follicle. Eggs are considered ready for release ("harvest") when the estrogen level starts to plateau and the sonogram shows two or more follicles, each with a mean diameter of eighteen millimeters. Follicles grow on the average of two to three millimeters per day. Exceedingly low levels of circulating estrogen are predictive of a poor response of the ovary, in which case the search for eggs by laparoscopy is likely to be fruitless.

The laparoscopic procedure is performed under light general anesthesia, and is timed to take place from thirty to thirty-four hours after hCG

Vitro Fertilization (New York: Springer-Verlag, 1984); M. Seppala and R. G. Edwards, eds., *In Vitro Fertilization and Embryo Transfer, Annals of the New York Academy of Sciences, Volume 442* (New York: The New York Academy of Sciences, 1985).

[6]The hormone hMG is rich in follicle-stimulating hormone (FSH) and is obtained from postmenopausal women. Even though FSH is no longer useful in the postmenopausal woman, it continues to be released by the pituitary gland. Although functionless, FSH accumulates in large quantities in the bloodstream of postmenopausal women.

[7]Ultrasound is a form of mechanical, vibrational energy whose frequency lies above the normal audible limit of 20,000 cycles per second. The pregnant uterus forms an excellent area for ultrasonic study. The sonic beam passes virtually intact through the amniotic fluid and sends back strong echoes from fetal and placental tissues. When the urinary bladder is filled, it acts as a water tank that permits the uterus itself to be well outlined. A woman in the *in vitro* clinic must have a full bladder before the ultrasound procedure, which entails drinking forty-eight ounces of fluid one-half hour before the appointment.

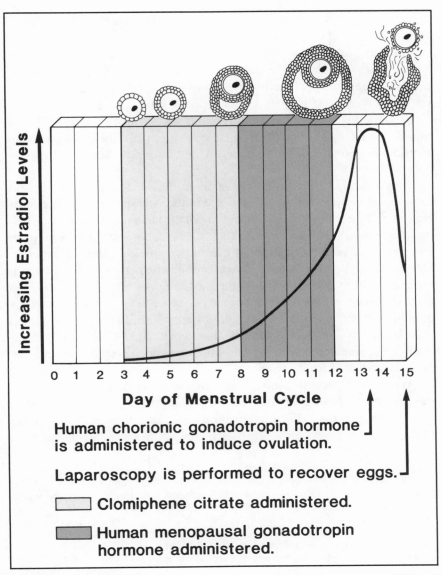

Chemically Induced Ovulation

Figure 8

Estrogen (estradiol) increases in response to chemical stimulation. When follicles mature (day thirteen), human gonadotropic hormone is administered to induce ovulation. Laparoscopy is performed thirty-six hours later to recover ripe eggs.

injection—as close as possible to the time of expected ovulation. Chemical stimulation of ovulation almost invariably results in the maturation of several fertilizable eggs. A number of large follicles are flushed, most of which typically yield fertilizable eggs. In some laboratories, ultrasound replaces or supplements laparoscopy in visualizing the mature follicles and retrieving the eggs (figure 9). Under local anesthesia, a needle is guided—along guidelines shown on the ultrasound scan—directly into the follicle to aspirate the egg. In contrast to laparoscopy, the ultrasound procedure requires only one abdominal puncture and does not necessitate general anesthesia.

The follicular aspirates are transported immediately to a culture laboratory usually located directly adjacent to the operating room. The fertilization of the egg and subsequent culture of the embryos require a carefully defined chemical solution ("medium"). The culture medium is prepared and tested for effectiveness about one to two weeks before laparoscopy. One way of testing the medium is to ascertain whether a sample will permit the growth of mouse embryos. If the medium does not promote development of mouse embryos to the blastocyst stage, the medium is unacceptable for human embryos. All conditions are carefully controlled, from a pH adjusted to 7.4 to a temperature maintained at 37°C. The culture medium is supplemented with serum, which had been prepared from blood obtained earlier from the patient.[8]

When the follicular aspirates are brought from the operating room to the laboratory, the eggs are immediately examined under a microscope for quality and maturity. The eggs are allowed to reach their peak of maturity in the culture medium for at least six hours before sperm are added.[9] The

---

[8]The commonly used chemical medium for fertilization is Ham's F10 media (Gibco Laboratories, Grand Island NY), which is reconstituted with distilled water and supplemented with calcium lactate, sodium bicarbonate, penicillin, and streptomycin. The medium is gassed with a mixture of 5% oxygen, 5% carbon dioxide, and 90% nitrogen, adjusted to a pH of 7.4 and supplemented with 15% serum. The medium in which the embryo is grown is slightly different, containing an HEPES buffer to maintain pH stability (Sigma Chemical Co., St. Louis MO) and a higher serum concentration (50%).

[9]Far-reaching experimentation on rabbit and hamster embryos served as the springboard for laboratory studies on the fertilization of human eggs. The first breakthrough came when M. C. Chang disclosed in 1959 (*Nature* 184:466-67) that rabbit eggs can be fertilized *in vitro*. Since that date, the successful fertilization of mammalian eggs in culture has been achieved in the mouse, cat, guinea pig, cow, baboon, chimpanzee, the Rhesus monkey, and the human, among others.

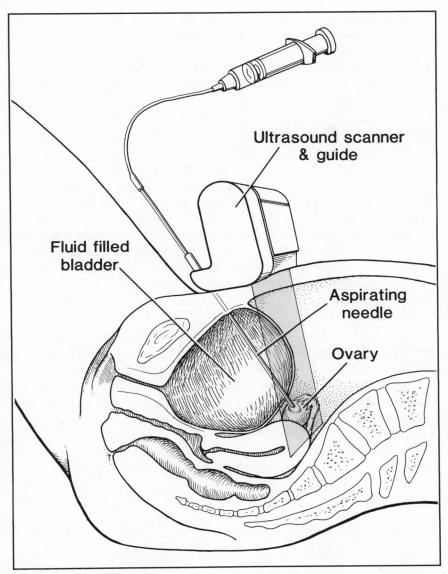

Retrieval of Eggs by Ultrasound **Figure 9**

A mature follicle is visualized by ultrasound, and the egg is aspirated by a needle that has been inserted by following the guidelines that are shown on the ultrasound scan.

semen of the husband is prepared for fertilization by several washings that remove inhibitory factors in the seminal fluid. The most motile sperm are segregated by a "swim-up" technique that favors the most active sperm. The sperm are allowed to swim up to the top of the medium in a plastic vial, and only the most active that succeed in reaching the top are selected. Normal semen has fifty- to seventy-percent motile sperm; the swim-up test yields a small, concentrated sample of about 200,000 sperm, of which ninety-five percent are highly motile.

Strange as it may seem, freshly ejaculated sperm cannot fertilize an egg. Sperm normally require a period of residence, or maturation, in the female genital tract. The subtle physiological changes by which a sperm cell acquires the ability to penetrate an egg has been termed *capacitation*. Investigators contemplating the technique of *in vitro* fertilization were aware of the poorly understood natural phenomenon of capacitation in humans. Fortuitously, it turns out that the chemical solutions used in preparing the suspension of sperm for *in vitro* fertilization somehow endows the sperm cell with the necessary properties to penetrate the egg. There is no evidence that failure of the sperm to pass through the female genital tract is associated with an increased risk of fertilization with abnormal sperm.[10]

The presence of two pronuclei—the male nuclear contribution from the sperm and the female nuclear contribution in the egg—signifies that fertilization has been achieved. The male and female pronuclei sit in close opposition to each other in the center of the egg (see figure 4 above). The pronuclei are usually visible from eighteen to twenty-two hours after the sperm has penetrated the egg. The fertilized eggs are critically examined for the presence of more than two pronuclei, which would signify that the egg had been penetrated by more than one sperm. Such eggs with supernumerary sperm nuclei rarely survive and, accordingly, are never knowingly implanted in the woman.[11]

---

[10]In normal circumstances, the passage of sperm through the female genital tract may be important in eliminating abnormal types of sperm. The "swim-up" test, which segregates the most motile sperm from the population, substitutes for the screening effect normally exerted by the female genital tract.

[11]When one sperm cell contacts the egg, changes occur in the zona pellucida (the thick outer coat surrounding the egg) that prevent the penetration of supernumerary sperm. Disfunction of this protective mechanism with the entry of more than one sperm leads to polyploidy (additional sets of chromosomes), which is generally lethal during early embryonic

The embryos are usually between the eight-cell and sixteen-cell stage when they are transferred nonsurgically to the woman. The woman is placed in a lithotomy (head-down tilt) position, which ensures that the path of the embryo to the uterus is downhill. The cervix is exposed with a speculum and the cervical mucus is gently wiped away with a dry swab. The transfer of the embryo is completed painlessly in a matter of minutes, and involves a specially designed catheter that is delivered into the cavity of the uterus through the cervix. After transfer of the embryo, the woman is kept at rest for four to eight hours, with the uterus in a dependent position. Shortly thereafter the woman is discharged from the hospital and advised to minimize physical activities for several days.

The woman is administered progesterone daily, either intramuscularly or in the form of a vaginal suppository, for at least two weeks to ensure a proper hormonal environment for implantation of the embryo. A pregnancy test is performed twelve days post-transfer and repeated twenty days post-transfer. Once pregnancy has been established, the pregnancy is monitored using all resources of the present state of the arts. The elaborate protocol includes continual office visits, hormonal analyses, ultrasound scan, serum α-fetoprotein testing (for spina bifida), amniocentesis (for prenatal biochemical and chromosomal analyses), routine obstetric laboratory tests, and two-hour postprandial glucose tests for signs of maternal diabetes.

Some couples go through the protocol several times. In most centers, a couple is usually not encouraged to go beyond three attempts. Every attempt at *in vitro* fertilization costs in the vicinity of $5,000 of which little, if any, is reimbursed by insurance coverage. A few insurance companies will pay for some of the services, such as laparoscopy and ultrasound. Other companies have refused to pay for any service on the grounds that reimbursement is made only for "clinically proven procedures." It is ironic that the *in vitro* fertilization procedure currently enjoys an overall success rate of pregnancy of at least twenty percent, which compares more favorably than the ten percent success rate of certain clinically proven heart operations that insurance companies cover unhesitatingly (figure 10).

The incidence of pregnancy increases with the transfer of more than one embryo. Whereas the success rate is cited at ten percent for the transfer

---

development. Polyploidy arises more often in immature oocytes, which suggests that the mechanisms for the prevention of polyspermic fertilization are relatively ineffective in immature oocytes.

**Embryos
implanted
naturally**

**Resulting
pregnancies**

30% Success rate

**Embryos
implanted
after in vitro
fertilization**

**Resulting
pregnancies**

20% Success rate

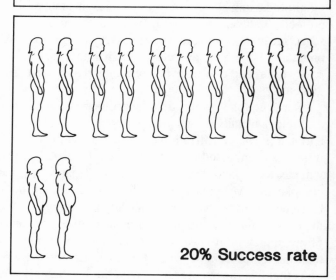

Success Rate of *in Vitro* Fertilization   **Figure 10**

Under optimum conditions normally, pregnancy is established for three out of ten embryos that implant in the uterus. The combination of superovulation and in vitro *fertilization yields a lower rate of pregnancy—two out of ten embryos that are transferred to the uterus.*

of one embryo, it is in excess of twenty percent when three embryos are implanted in a given trial. Not more than three embryos are generally transplanted to the uterus because of the obstetric risks associated with the potential establishment of multiple pregnancies, particularly quadruplet pregnancies, as well as the potential for ectopic (abnormally positioned) pregnancies. If more than three eggs are recovered from the ovary by laparoscopy, the thorny question arises as to the dispersal of the excess eggs. Several options may be considered. Not all recovered eggs need be fertilized, thereby limiting the number of embryos to the exact number to be implanted. On the other hand, all eggs can be fertilized and the excess embryos can be frozen for subsequent use in another trial at a later date. One may also consider the possibility of donating the extra eggs to a recipient woman who is medically unable to produce her own eggs. It is glaringly apparent that these varied options are accompanied by a whole range of new and unprecedented moral dilemmas.

Chapter 4

Expectations and Risks

During the 1970s, there was genuine anxiety about the unforeseen risks to the embryo of the *in vitro* fertilization procedures. At the time, the uneasiness was over whether intervention into the normal reproductive process might result in a deformed child. The issue could not then be addressed because of the dearth of information from research or clinical trials. Today, the widespread clinical application of *in vitro* fertilization has done much to dispel many of the nagging concerns. The evidence is clear that the embryo is not subject to extraordinary hazards. There has been no discernible increase in the incidence of congenital defects or in neonatal mortality among the products of *in vitro* fertilization.

The *in vitro* studies are best evaluated in light of what is presently known of normal events in embryonic development. Most people do not realize that the rate of embryo loss in naturally occurring pregnancies is very high. Two in every three conceptuses are aborted involuntarily, so it is not unusual for any woman to have had a spontaneous abortion—unknowingly or knowingly.[1] This astonishing statement may be better understood if we explore what happens to twenty eggs produced by women who are reproducing naturally (figure 11). Under conditions optimal for fertilization, three of the twenty eggs will fail to be fertilized. In other words, after ex-

---

[1]H. Leridon, *Human Fertility: The Basic Components* (Chicago: University of Chicago Press, 1977).

Test-Tube Conception

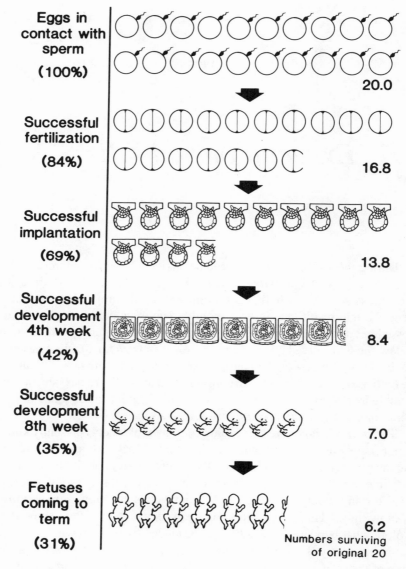

Eggs in contact with sperm (100%) — 20.0

Successful fertilization (84%) — 16.8

Successful implantation (69%) — 13.8

Successful development 4th week (42%) — 8.4

Successful development 8th week (35%) — 7.0

Fetuses coming to term (31%) — 6.2

Numbers surviving of original 20

Pregnancy Wastage

Figure 11

For a typical woman with normal ovulation in which twenty eggs are released over a period of time, only six of the twenty eggs (thirty-one percent) can be expected to result in a pregnancy with the delivery of a livebirth.

posure to sperm, the probability of fertilization of an egg is eighty-four percent. Of the seventeen eggs that are fertilized, three will fail to implant. Of the fourteen embryos implanted at the end of the first week, six of these characteristically will find the uterine lining inhospitable. Thus, only eight eggs of the original twenty are of such viability as to cause the woman to miss her expected menstrual period. Stated another way, by the time pregnancy is recognizable, more than half the eggs have been lost. At eight weeks' gestation when the embryo is now termed a fetus, thirteen eggs of the original twenty will have failed to survive. Fortunately, the incidence of spontaneous abortion occurring at some point during eight to twenty-eight weeks' gestation is very low. By the end of the gestation period, about one-third of all fertilizable eggs manage to develop to term. Thus, for a typical woman with normal ovulation, a pregnancy with the delivery of a livebirth can be expected only with a probability of thirty-one percent.[2]

What accounts for the high incidence of naturally occurring, or spontaneous, abortions in humans? Studies of spontaneous human abortuses have revealed that the major cause of embryonic and fetal loss is faulty, or abnormal, chromosomes. As high as fifty percent of the human embryos that implant successfully have chromosome abnormalities that endanger their chances of survival.[3] The most common abnormalities include the presence of an additional chromosome, such as an extra twenty-first chro-

---

[2]Demographers employ a different mathematical approach in evaluating a woman's fecundity—that is, the probability of conception during a given month resulting in a livebirth. The analysis shows that about four months of sexual activity are necessary for fifty percent of the women to become pregnant, and eight months for seventy percent to become pregnant. See J. Bongaarts, "A Method for the Estimation of Fecundability," *Demography* 12 (1975): 645-60. These figures can be adapted for the *in vitro* fertilization process in which a single embryo is recovered and implanted. The *in vitro* fertilization procedure would have to be repeated four times for pregnancy to occur in fifty percent of the women, and eight times for success in seventy percent of the women. See J. D. Biggers, "*In Vitro* Fertilization and Embryo Transfer in Human Beings," *New England Journal of Medicine* 304 (1981): 336-42.

[3]Most of the chromosomally abnormal embryos perish in the first trimester of pregnancy. Between the second and seventh week of pregnancy, sixty-six of the 100 abortuses have abnormal chromosomes. The incidence of chromosome anomalies falls to twenty-three among 100 abortuses between eight to twelve weeks of age. By the end of the second trimester, the frequency of chromosomal abnormalities in spontaneous abortions decreases from more than eighty percent in the early stages of pregnancy to less than five percent. See J. Boué and A. Boué, "Chromosomal Anomalies in Early Spontaneous Abortion," *Current Topics in Pathology* 62 (1976): 193-205.

mosome that causes Down syndrome, and the absence of an X chromosome in the female that causes Turner syndrome. Some of the conceptuses may have a complete extra set of chromosomes, an abnormal state known as triploidy. The presence of abnormal complements of chromosomes usually prevents the embryos from developing to term. In essence, the normal reproductive processes in humans are characterized by a high incidence of embryonic deaths associated with faulty chromosomes.[4]

The age of the woman has strong bearing on the rate of spontaneous abortions and the frequency of chromosomal abnormalities. Women between twenty and twenty-four years of age have the least risk for spontaneously aborting their offspring (sixteen per one-hundred pregnancies), while women between thirty-five and thirty-nine years have the greatest risk (thirty-seven per one-hundred pregnancies). The frequency of chromosomal abnormalities in the offspring also increases with maternal age.[5] As a specific example, the incidence of Down syndrome increases markedly with the age of the mother, occurring about one in 1,600 births at maternal age twenty to one in 100 births at age forty. Among women over forty-five, one in forty infants may be expected to be affected with Down syndrome.

It may be disconcerting to learn that there is a large natural loss of embryos in pregnancy. The important point, however, is the high efficiency with which nature eliminates abnormal embryos during the course of pregnancy. For every 1,000 chromosomal abnormalities that are present in the womb, only six are expected to survive to the point of a livebirth. Thus,

---

[4]Most chromosomal imbalances arise during the maturation (meiosis) of the egg or sperm cell. The process of maturation of the gametes is complex and subject to error. Occasional accidents occur in the bahavior of chromosomes such that an egg (or sperm) comes to contain both members of a given pair of chromosomes, instead of the usual one member of a given pair. For example, such a mishap (technically, "nondisjunction") involving the 21st pair of chromosomes would result in an egg cell that possesses two 21st chromosomes instead of the customary one. This egg cell, when fertilized by a normal sperm, would produce a Down infant that has three 21st chromosomes. The Down infant is said to be "trisomic" for the 21st chromosome.

[5]Chromosome abnormalities have been shown to be related to repetitive, or habitual, abortions. Some couples have a tendency to have repeated spontaneous abortions because they produce chromosomally abnormal gametes. For example, if the first abortus is trisomic, the likelihood is about eighty percent that the second will also be trisomic. See T. Kaji and A. Ferrier, "Cytogenetics of Abortuses," *American Journal of Obstetrics and Gynecology* 131 (1978): 33.

99.4 percent of the chromosomal abnormalities are eliminated naturally through spontaneous abortion. To cite a specific case, ninety-five percent of conceptuses with Turner syndrome are spontaneously aborted. Nature has created a great barrier to the perpetuation of the chromosomally abnormal offspring. Nature, however, is not perfect. Some chromosomally abnormal fetuses escape nature's screening mechanism and survive to term. Down syndrome represents one of nature's failures; only eighty percent of Down infants are aborted spontaneously. About twenty percent go on to be liveborn.

With the advent of prenatal diagnosis, parents have been afforded the opportunity of ameliorating nature's shortcomings by averting the births of demonstrably abnormal fetuses. It bears emphasizing that the thrust of prenatal diagnosis is to prevent the tragic impact of serious chromosomal (and biochemical) disorders. Chromosomal abnormalities can be diagnosed *in utero* at approximately sixteen weeks' gestation by a procedure known as amniocentesis (figure 12). The procedure involves the removal of a sample of the fluid in the amniotic cavity surrounding the developing fetus. Cells are continually shed into the amniotic fluid and these free floating cells have been shown to be of fetal origin. They can be grown in laboratory cultures to preview the chromosomes. Amniocentesis has been done primarily on limited groups of women who are at high risk of bearing a chromosomally abnormal child, such as women over thirty-five. Today, amniocentesis is routinely offered at *in vitro* clinics.

We may now inquire as to whether the technique of *in vitro* fertilization imposes a greater risk than usual that the implanted embryo will abort or be born defective. We have seen that 99.4 percent of the chromosomal abnormalities in embryos are eliminated naturally through spontaneous abortion. We can reasonably expect a comparable elimination of abnormal embryos in pregnant women utilizing the *in vitro* technique. The existing data indicate that the vast majority of chromosomally abnormal embryos are eliminated in early pregnancy, as occurs under normal conditions.[6] The expectation is also that some, although relatively few, chromosomally aberrant embryos will survive to term, as also occurs naturally. In fact, in early 1985, a child with Down syndrome was born to a twenty-eight-year-

---

[6]R. R. Angell, R. J. Aitken, P. F. A. van Look, M. A. Lumsden, and A. A. Templeton, "Chromosome Abnormalities in Human Embryos After *in Vitro* Fertilization," *Nature* 303 (1983): 326-38.

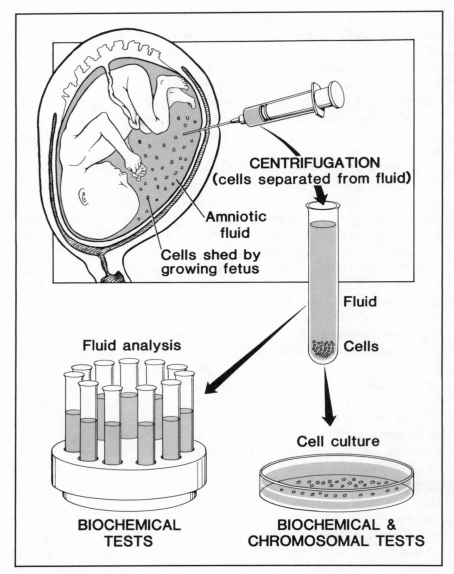

Technique of Amniocentesis   **Figure 12**

A small sample of amniotic fluid is withdrawn by inserting a needle through the abdomen into the uterine cavity at fourteen to sixteen weeks of pregnancy. The amniotic fluid contains fetal cells which can be analyzed for biochemical and chromosomal fetal disorders.

old woman at an *in vitro* clinic in Houston.[7] This case is of special interest in that the woman did not avail herself of amniocentesis because she was reluctant to accept even the small risk of fetal loss that amniocentesis entails.[8]

The more incisive question is whether any phase of the *in vitro* fertilization procedure will foster or promote chromosomal abnormalities, so as to increase the risk of birth defects above the natural level. It has been suggested that the ovulation-inducing drugs (clomiphene and/or hMG) might trigger increased chromosomal aberrations, but such a supposition has yet to be verified.[9] There is also the unconfirmed hypothesis that polyspermy might occur more often because the concentrations of sperm used *in vitro* exceed the known concentrations of sperm in the upper reaches of the fallopian tube at natural conception.[10] Even if an increased risk of polyspermy were the case, it is highly unlikely that the resulting embryos would

---

[7]J. F. Hejtmancik, D. H. Ledbetter, A. L. Beaudet, and M. M. Quigley, "A Trisomic Child After *in Vitro* Fertilization: Result of Paternal Nondisjunction," *Fertility and Sterility* 44 (1985): 830-31.

[8]The findings of several studies indicate that amniocentesis is a safe and highly accurate procedure that does not significantly increase the risk of fetal injury or loss. Given the high rate of naturally occurring abortion, it is difficult to demonstrate unequivocally that a spontaneous abortion after amniocentesis is a direct consequence of the procedure. The question that can be answered is whether fetal loss occurs more often after amniocentesis than usual. Statistically, there is no demonstrable increased risk of abortion following amniocentesis. In a large sample in the United Staes, 3.5 percent of pregnant women who underwent amniocentesis experienced fetal loss subsequent to the procedure. But the frequency in control subjects is 3.2 percent; the difference between 3.2 and 3.5 is not statistically significant. See NICHD Registry for Amniocentesis Study Group, "Midtrimester Amniocentesis for Prenatal Diagnosis: Safety and Accuracy," *Journal of the Medical Association* 236 (1976): 1471-76.

[9]J. G. Boué and A. Boué, "Increased Frequency of Chromosomal Anomalies in Abortions After Induced Ovulation," *Lancet* 1 (1973): 679-80; N. Laufer, B. M. Pratt, A. H. DeCherney, F. Naftolin, et al., "The *in Vivo* and *in Vitro* Effects of Clomiphene Citrate on Ovulation, Fertilization, and Development of Cultural Mouse Oocytes," *American Journal of Obstetrics and Gynecology* 147 (1983): 633-39.

[10]L. R. Fraser, H. M. Zanellotti, and G. R. Paton. "Increased Incidence of Triploidy in Embryos Derived from Mouse Eggs Fertilized in Vitro," *Nature* 260 (1976): 39-40; I. Maudlin and L. R. J. Fraser, "The Effect of PMSG Dose on the Incidence of Chromosomal Anomalies in Mouse Embryos Fertilized in Vitro," *Journal of Reproduction and Fertility* 50 (1977): 275-80; T. Asakawa and W. R. Kukelow, "Chromosomal Analyses After *in Vitro* Fertilization of Squirrel Monkey (*Saimiri Sciureus*) Oocytes," *Biology of Reproduction* 26 (1982): 579-83.

develop to term. Some investigators have claimed, with scarcely any sub-
stantiation, that fertilization of the egg *in vitro* may be associated with an
increased risk of fertilization with abnormal sperm, inasmuch as the sperm
population has not been screened for abnormal types by the usual passage
through the female genital tract.[11]

On the other hand, one could argue that *fewer* chromosomal abnormalities might be anticipated in babies born following *in vitro* fertilization.
There is appreciable evidence that chromosomal aberrations frequently arise
when eggs are fertilized at the close of their life span.[12] Eggs that experience a delay in insemination are said to be "aged" or "overripe." Since
sexual activity in humans is not restricted to the precise moment of ovulation, a certain percentage of eggs are likely to be fertilized two or three
days after ovulation. With *in vitro* fertilization, ovulation and insemination are so precisely synchronized that the risk of fertilization of an overripe, or aged, egg is appreciably diminished, if not virtually eliminated.

Overall, there appears to be little, if any, danger of increased congenital defects from the *in vitro* procedure.[13] Admittedly, the number of infants born is insufficient to rule out some degree of increased (or decreased)
risk, even to liveborn offspring. From a statistical standpoint, the extent
of risk must remain an open question. Even a *large* increase in the per-
centages of abnormal embryos that might theoretically result from the *in
vitro* procedure would show up only as a *very small* increase in the number
of affected infants. The impressive mathematical considerations of Dr. J.

---

[11]J. W. Overstreet and D. F. Katz, "Sperm Transport and Selection in the Female Genital Tract," *Development in Mammals,* Vol. 2, ed. M. H. Johnson (Amsterdam: North-
Holland, 1977): 31-65.

[12]By experimentally delaying the time of insemination of rabbit eggs, the British biologist C. R. Austin established that at least fifty percent of the overripe eggs met early death
before they ever began implanting in the uterus. In guinea pigs and cattle, aging of eggs is
associated with a high incidence of abortion and stillbirths. Apparently, for best chances
of fertilization as well as better chances of normal development, sperm should lie in wait
for the egg so that the meeting of the two takes place soon after ovulation. See C. R. Austin,
"Chromosome Deterioration in Aging Eggs of the Rabbit," *Nature* 213 (1967) 1018-19.

[13]I. Craft, F. McLeod, S. Green, et al., "Human Pregnancy Following Oocyte and Sperm
Transfer to the Uterus," *Lancet* 1 (1982) 1031-33; H. W. Jones, Jr., "The Ethics of *in
Vitro* Fertilization," *Fertility and Sterility* 37 (1982): 146-49.

J. Schlesselman[14] show that if the frequency of chromosomal abnormalities were to be increased twofold by the *in vitro* technique, it would require a sample size of about 1,000 infants to detect such an increase with reasonable reliability. What can be stated definitively at this time is that well over 1,000 infants have already been born, and we have yet to witness even a modicum of increase, either in the number or type of chromosomal abnormality.

The overwhelming majority of infants born from *in vitro* procedures have been free from major defects. Indeed, the exceptionally good results could have been anticipated in light of the premium status applied to *in vitro* pregnancies. The pregnancies have been carefully monitored to curtail all potential hazards, even to the point of affecting delivery by caesarean section to avoid the hazards of labor. In fact, such great status or value has been placed on *in vitro* babies that the expression "premium babies" has been coined.[15] The follow-up studies of some of the children, extending almost to the early school years, have been gratifying. Neither the physical nor mental development of the children has been impaired in any way.[16]

---

[14]For the sake of argument, let us assume that the treatment associated with *in vitro* fertilization does enhance the survival of naturally occurring chromosomal abnormalities. A *marked* increase in the frequency of chromosomal abnormalities at implantation is expected to have only a *minor* effect on the frequency of abnormalities among livebirths. Since only 0.6 percent of the abnormalities at implantation occur in fetuses that survive to the point of livebirth, a twofold increase in the frequency of abnormalities at implantation would result in only two to three additional abnormalities per 1,000 livebirths. From a statistical point of view, the additional abnormalities would scarcely be evident. See J. J. Schlesselman, "How Does One Assess the Risk of Abnormalities from Human *in Vitro* Fertilization?", *American Journal of Obstetrics and Gynecology* 135 (1979): 135-48.

[15]L. Karp, "Premium babies," *American Journal of Medical Genetics* 12 (1982): 369-70.

[16]The fears that the *in vitro* child in later life might show abnormalities seem groundless. A priori, normal neonatal development is predictable from studies of babies born following artificial insemination by husband (A.I.H) or artificial insemination by donor (A.I.D.). The development of these children compares favorably with the average child in the general population. See R. Zizuka, Y. Sawada, N. Nishira, and M. Ohi, "The Physical and Mental Development of Children Born Following Artificial Insemination," *International Journal of Fertility* 13 (1968): 24-32.

Chapter 5

Moral Status of the Embryo

The efficacy of the *in vitro* fertilization procedure is noticeably increased by retrieving several preovulatory eggs from the mother. To enhance the chance of a favorable pregnancy outcome, most clinics customarily remove several preovulatory eggs from the prospective mother. When only two or three of several artificially fertilized eggs are implanted, who decides what is to be done with the surplus embryos? Are the extra embryos to be used for research? Or are they to be destroyed? If the surplus embryos are discarded, then human embryonic development is deliberately initiated with the certain knowledge that the life of several embryos will not be sustained. On the other hand, if the extra embryos are abnormal, does the physician avert accusation for destroying life by implanting the abnormal embryos in the woman, secure in the knowledge that aberrant embryos have little chance for survival in the uterus?

At the heart of the problem is the profound question as to when the human embryo should enjoy the same moral status as a child or an adult. The opinion has been forcibly voiced by Paul Ramsey and others[1] that the embryo warrants dignity, if not protection of the law, because of its potential to become a fully developed human being. It follows that the destruction

---

[1] P. Ramsey, "Shall We 'Reproduce'? I. The Medical Ethics of *in Vitro* Fertilization," *Journal of the American Medical Association* 220 (1972): 1346-50; H. O. Tiefel, "Human *in Vitro* Fertilization: A Conservative View," *Journal of the American Medical Association* 247 (1982): 3235-42.

or experimental manipulation of an embryo is morally repugnant because it would deny the opportunity for the embryo to realize its potential. This view is deserving of thoughtful exploration.[2]

The continuity of life is assured by reproduction, the process by which an organism leaves descendants. The essential feature of sexual reproduction is that each parent contributes to its offspring only a single specialized sex cell, either an egg or sperm cell. These two minute sex cells, or gametes, are the only physical bridge between the parents and offspring. The offspring begins its existence the moment that the sperm nucleus unites with the egg nucleus. The new individual is endowed with a unique package of inherited units, or genes, which direct development and growth in a specific way. In other words, the individual is endowed with a genetic code that deals with all the traits the individual will show. Indeed, the genetic code for each human zygote is unique. Except for possible mutational changes, the code established in the zygote is the same thirty years later and, in fact, until the individual dies. Viewed in this manner, the *biological* life of each human being traces back to the fertilized egg when this new cell acquires a unique genetic package.[3]

Although biological life may be viewed as commencing at fertilization, the fertilized egg is scarcely more than the blueprints for a human being. Stated another way, the genetic code of a zygote is not actually a human being, just as a set of blueprints is not really a house. Thus, conception only establishes the *potentiality* for human existence. One could now contend that it would be morally wrong to create new life with the potential for becoming a human being and then deliberately destroy it or use it in experimentation. Accordingly, advocates of this view hold that the human embryo should be given special protection so that its potential

---

[2]The literature is replete with articles on the intrinsic value of early human life. Some thoughtful discussions and literature citations may be found in the following books: C. Grobstein, *From Chance to Purpose* (London: Addison-Wesley Publishing Company, 1981); W. A. W. Walters and P. Singer, eds., *Test-Tube Babies* (New York: Oxford University Press, 1982); M. W. Shaw and A. E. Doudera, eds., *Defining Human Life* (Ann Arbor, AUPHA Press, 1983).

[3]This view is not necessarily conclusive. To assert that life begins at conception is to suggest that what existed before the zygote is not life. On the contrary, the sperm cell before fertilization and the unfertilized egg cell are very much alive. See H. W. Jones, Jr., "The Ethics of *in Vitro* Fertilization—1981," *Human Conception in Vitro*, R. G. Edwards and J. M. Purdy, eds. (New York: Academic Press, 1982) 351-57.

may be fulfilled.[4] In particular, since *in vitro* fertilization makes the early embryo accessible to manipulation in a culture dish, special protection is sought for the preimplantation embryo—before it has imbedded in the uterine wall of the mother.

If the embryo is entitled to protection, then it must be granted the status of personhood and afforded human rights. The incisive issue, then, is whether and at what stage the developing embryo exists as a person with human rights. In essence, the core question is: When is personhood conferred in humans?[5]

The human embryo, at present, has no legal status as a person. When the Supreme Court held in *Roe v. Wade* that the constitutionally protected right of privacy encompasses a woman's decision to terminate pregnancy, it rejected the argument that the word ''person'' in the Fourteenth Amendment included the unborn. Hence, it denied the embryo (and fetus) a claim to constitutional rights equal to that of the pregnant woman. In essence, the assumption implicit in the legalization of abortion is that the embryo is far from being a person.[6]

Right-to-life advocates believe that the Supreme Court was mistaken and misguided in their landmark decision. Senator Jesse A. Helms, a fundamentalist from North Carolina, has tried, in vain, to persuade Congress to pass a constitutional amendment that would extend constitutional pro-

---

[4]Not every fertilized human egg has the potential for being a human being. All molar, or hydatidiform, pregnancies (which contain no evidence of an embryo) are the result of fertilization and are genetically unique. Conversely, some teratomas have some of the characteristics of a new individual but are not the result of the union of sperm and egg.

[5]The companion question as to when ''personhood'' begins is the equally elusive query as to when ''ensoulment'' takes place—the moment when the soul (a quality unique only to humans among animals) enters the embryo. The Catholic tradition has unhesitatingly endowed the fertilized egg with an everlasting soul. If ensoulment occurs at fertilization, then special provision must be made for monozygotic twins since the twinning process occurs much later than fertilization.

[6]On 22 January 1973, the United States Supreme Court enunciated in *Roe v. Wade,* that ''we need not resolve the difficult question of when life begins. When those trained in the respective disciplines of medicine, philosophy and theology are unable to arrive at any consensus, the judiciary, at this point in the development of man's knowledge, is not in a position to speculate as to the answer.'' U.S. Supreme Court, *Roe v. Wade,* 410 U.S. 113 (1973).

tection to the embryo from the moment of conception.[7] When it became apparent that such an amendment would fail to obtain the two-thirds majority needed in both houses of Congress, some right-to-life advocates, led by Helms, tried to circumvent the constitutional amendment vote by urging Congress to pass, by a simple majority vote, the so-called Human Life Bill.[8] The Bill contained the declaration that a fetus is a person under the Fourteenth Amendment. This Bill, and various versions thereafter, failed to gain passage in Congress.

There seems to have emerged a consensus that the human embryo is entitled to profound respect, but this respect does not encompass the legal rights attributed to persons.[9] The early embryo is not upheld as a person because, more often than not, it does not realize its biologic potential. The potential is merely statistical, since only about one in three human zygotes normally reaches term successfully (see discussion in chapter 4). Even though the embryo is not accorded the status equivalent to that of a person, the medical profession acknowledges its traditional obligation of avoiding risks of known harm to the embryo. For the medical practitioner, life is a continuum which ethics and the law vainly strive to divide at arbitrary points. It is unfathomable to ask a physician to refrain from applying medical knowledge to early embryonic life. Almost on a daily basis, physicians are called upon to apply the most modern medical technology to

---

[7]Senator Helm's Human Life Amendment (2038) to debt ceiling legislation in 1981 included the following declarations: "The Congress finds that . . . scientific evidence demonstrates that the life of each individual begins at conception; . . . the Supreme Court . . . erred in not recognizing the humanity of the unborn child and the compelling interest of the several states in protecting the life of each person before birth, and . . . in excluding unborn children from the safeguards afforded by the equal protection provisions of the Constitution."

[8]Helms-Hyde Human Life Bill, S. 158, 97th Congress, 1st Session (1981). This bill and other "human life" statutes were expressly drafted to ban or limit the availability of abortions indirectly by broadening the definition of "person" to include the embryo. Most legal authorities have voiced the opinion that the appropriate way to address the abortion issue is through the vehicle of a constitutional amendment dealing directly with abortion, and not by prescribing that the conceptus is a person. See D. Westfall, "Beyond Abortion: The Potential Reach of the Human Life Amendment." *American Journal of Law and Medicine* 8 (1982): 97-135.

[9]D. M. Flannery, C. D. Weisman, C. R. Lipsett, and A. N. Braverman, "Test-Tube Babies: Legal Issues Raised by in Vitro Fertilization," *Georgetown Law Journal* 67(1979): 1295-1304.

diagnose and treat diseases at various stages in one's life. If it is permissible to alleviate disease during childhood or adulthood, would it not also be permissible to ameliorate disease during early embryonic life? If the embryo were to be conferred personhood, physicians would be defenseless in extending their diagnostic prowess to the embryo.

The diagnosis of disease in early embryonic life becomes a particularly important consideration in terms of our current understanding of inherited disorders. Genetically transmissible disorders contribute substantially to human ill health, including severe mental retardation. Reliable estimates indicate that one of every eight pediatric hospital beds today is occupied by a child with a congenital disorder in which hereditary factors play a prominent role. There is little that can be done to prevent most inherited abnormalities from expressing their crippling effects once the child is delivered. The advent of prenatal diagnosis in the 1960s permitted the detection of several genetic diseases while the fetus is still developing in the uterus.

Until recently, pediatricians were limited in their capacity to determine if an expectant mother might deliver a child with a serious birth defect. For the most part, pediatricians referred prospective parents with a family history of a congenital disorder to specialists in genetic counseling. Even then the prospective parents could be informed only of the statistical probability that they would have a child with a particular congenital disorder. No assurance could be given that the actual outcome of the pregnancy would not be unfavorable.[10] Many high-risk couples in the past avoided pregnancy rather than hazard the birth of a defective child. Today, prenatal diagnosis of fetal abnormalities through amniocentesis or chorionic villus sampling remains the most valuable option for the avoidance of serious or fatal birth defects. The fundamental philosophy of prenatal diagnosis is to provide an option for parents at risk to avert the birth of a defective child by elective abortion of demonstrably affected fetuses.[11]

---

[10]Most babies with inherited disorders are born to couples without prior warning. Many faulty genes are recessive, causing a disorder when present in double dose in an individual. Thus, the malfunctioning gene must be inherited from both parents for the disease to occur in the offspring. A person who has only one faulty copy will not ordinarily develop the symptoms of the disease but will be a carrier. There are many more unaffected carrier parents of a recessive trait than there are individuals manifesting the recessive disorder.

[11]It should be clear that no woman subjects herself to an abortion unless she feels she

Any legislation defining the embryo or fetus as a person would have a profoundly negative impact on the progress achieved in recent years in prenatal diagnosis. Such legislation would declare rights for the conceptus equal to those of the mother who is carrying that conceptus. Mother and fetus would no longer be viewed as a single entity sharing harmonious interests but rather as two distinct patients. The interests of the two "persons" in one body would certainly conflict. One of the most devastating genetic disorders is the inherited condition known as Tay-Sachs disease, which dooms the infant to a lingering and painful death, usually by age four.[12] Such a trauma understandably causes a couple to seek an absolute guarantee against the recurrence of Tay-Sachs in a subsequent pregnancy. With legislation establishing fetal personhood, the genetic screening program designed to offer the option of abortion in instances of a second unfavorable pregnancy would be of no benefit, since the woman could be denied the choice of therapeutic abortion. Clearly, women at genetic risk would avoid a subsequent pregnancy, as they had before the advent of prenatal diagnosis. It should be underscored that many women with genetic risk now undertake pregnancies only because of the availability of prenatal diagnosis. In this respect, prenatal diagnosis may be viewed as birth-facilitating rather than birth-preventing. Stated another way, the availability of prenatal diagnosis, particularly for the older woman, makes conception acceptable where previously it was often avoided because of the risk, even when small, of bearing an affected child.

Medicine's ability to treat fetal defects has achieved considerable sophistication. Dramatic progress has been made in extending surgical procedures to the developing fetus in the womb. In certain disorders, the specific malformation in the fetus not only can be recognized *in utero*, but can be treated *in utero*.[13] In a Denver hospital in 1981, surgeons have re-

---

must. Most women who have an abortion do not regard it as "just another" surgical treatment. Abortion remains, at the least, an unpleasant experience. If one takes the absolutist position that abortion is morally indefensible under any circumstance, then prenatal diagnosis aimed at the selective elimination of genetically abnormal fetuses can have no place in medical practice. Certainly those who adhere to the absolutist position will themselves avoid abortion and hopefully not condemn those who condone it.

[12]An entire chapter is devoted to Tay-Sachs disease in a monograph by the present author (E. Peter Volpe) in *Patient in the Womb* (Macon GA: Mercer University Press, 1984).

[13]M. R. Harrison, R. A. Filly, J. T. Parer, et al., "Management of the Fetus with a Urinary Tract Malfunction," *Journal of the American Medical Association* 246 (1981): 635-39; and M. R. Harrison, M. S. Golbus, R. A. Filly, et al., "Fetal Surgery for Congenital Hydronephrosis," *New England Journal of Medicine* 306 (1982): 591-93.

lieved pressure from the brain of a hydrocephalic fetus by implanting a small valve into the skull of the fetus. In the same year in San Francisco, a team of physicians successfully operated on a congenitally obstructed urinary tract in one of a pair of unborn twins. A newly designed catheter was skill-fully guided through the wall of the mother's abdomen, through the uterus, and into the distended bladder of the affected fetus. The catheter was re-moved at birth, and the previously affected male twin, while requiring fur-ther corrective surgery, is expected to be as normal as his sister.

At present, a woman has the unrestricted right to refuse to consent to surgery for her unborn child. But the situation would change strikingly if the fetus were legally a person with the same rights as the woman. If there is a conflict between the interests of the woman and those of the fetus, who would speak on behalf of the fetus? Should a doctor be liable for damages if he prevents the death of a fetus by surgery *in utero,* but the fetus is born severely damaged? If a woman is carrying a multiple pregnancy in which one fetus is abnormal, is the physician justified in endangering the normal fetus in an effort to treat the abnormal one? The ethical issues surrounding fetal surgery are complicated enough without introducing another poi-gnant variable by conferring personhood on the fetus.

Just as the fetus has become the subject for medical therapy, it seems likely that the embryo will attain the status of a patient. As indicated ear-lier, a certain proportion of embryos will be carrying faulty genes. On what basis would it be considered improper or unethical to monitor or detect these abnormal genes in early embryonic life? If we could monitor for the pres-ence of an abnormal gene in early embryos, then by the use of *in vitro* fer-tilization, it would be possible to ensure that only normal embryos are implanted in the mother, particularly in those families in which there are carriers of serious genetic disorders.

In like manner, infertile couples who are at risk of transmitting a chro-mosome anomaly could be assured that the implanted embryos are chro-mosomally normal. Chromosomal abnormalities do occur with high frequencies in human conceptuses that are produced by *in vitro* fertiliza-tion, as they do in embryos produced naturally. The chromosome consti-tution of the embryo can be established from cytological analyses of but a few cells. Roslyn Angell and her colleagues at the University of Edinburgh have described a method of examining chromosomes in eight-cell human embryos.[14] Accordingly, the possibility exists of determining the chromosome makeup of an eight-celled or sixteen-celled conceptus by removing one or two of its cells and culturing them for chromosomal analysis. The conceptus in the meantime would be frozen and afterwards thawed out and transferred to the woman only if the cells were shown to be normal. Lest one be concerned about the loss of one or two cells, it has already been shown that a frozen eight-celled mammalian conceptus that has lost some of its cells can give rise to a normal fetus.[15] As the molecular techniques become more sophisticated, the cell removed from the early embryo can be assessed not only for chromosomal aberrations, but for certain defective genes that cause debilitating malformations.

A cell removed from an early embryo can be critically analyzed for malfunctioning genes by employing modern techniques devised by molecular geneticists. As presently understood, a gene is a coded sequence of the DNA molecule in the nucleus of the cell.[16] The search for a defective gene begins by using a special class of enzymes, called *restriction enzymes,* that fragment the long DNA strand at several points. These enzymes act as chemical scissors; they cut the DNA strand at precise sites.

A gene is responsible for specifying the production of a particular protein, such as the hemoglobin molecule. A particular restriction enzyme is capable of recognizing the coding sequence of the normal gene that directs the chemical pattern of hemoglobin. Hence, in a person with the normal protein, the fragment of DNA associated with the normal gene has a characteristic length (figure 13). If a mutation were to occur that alters the

---

[14]R. R. Angell, R. J. Aitken, P. F. A. van Look, M. A. Lumsden, and A. A. Templeton, "Chromosome Abnormalities in Human Embryos After *in Vitro* Fertilization," *Nature* 303 (1983): 336-38.

[15]A. McLaren, "The Embryo," *Reproduction in Mammals: Embryonic and Fetal Development,* ed. C. R. Austin and R. V. Short (Cambridge: Cambridge University Press, 1982) 1-25.

[16]One of the finest triumphs of modern science has been the elucidation of the chemical nature of the gene. The transmission of traits from parents to offspring depends on the transfer of a specific giant molecule that carries a coded blueprint in its molecular structure. This complex molecule, the basic chemical component of the chromosome, is *deoxyribonucleic acid,* often referred to in its abbreviated form, DNA. The information carried in this molecule can be divided into a number of separable units, now recognized as the genes. Stated simply, chromosomes are primarily long strands of DNA, and genes are coded sequences of the DNA molecule. The amount of DNA present in a single unfertilized human egg has been estimated to carry information corresponding to two million genes.

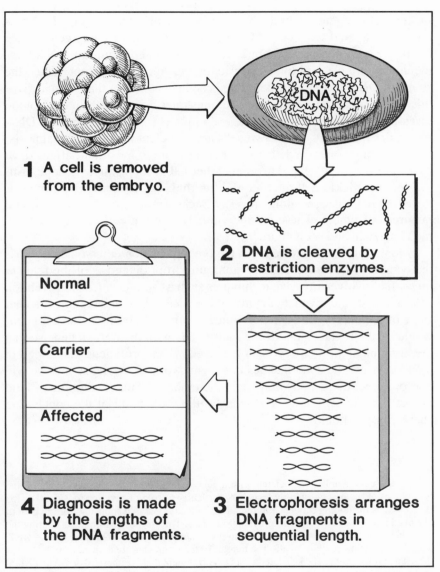

1 A cell is removed from the embryo.

2 DNA is cleaved by restriction enzymes.

Normal

Carrier

Affected

4 Diagnosis is made by the lengths of the DNA fragments.

3 Electrophoresis arranges DNA fragments in sequential length.

Molecular Diagnosis of Genetic Disorders   **Figure 13**

Restriction enzymes cleave the DNA strands, and electrophoretic techniques sort out the DNA so that the fragments can be identified by length.

makeup of the gene, then the restriction enzyme would be unable to recognize the altered sequence of DNA associated with the faulty gene. Since the faulty gene does not generate the same normal protein, the DNA fragments that are cleaved by the restriction enzyme are different. Thus, the strand of DNA carrying the defective gene may be longer than normal. That this actually can occur has been demonstrated for the debilitating blood disease, sickle cell anemia.[17] The technique is so sensitive that the DNA molecules from only one or two cells are sufficient to make the diagnosis. By this means, one can detect whether the embryo is normal, affected, or a carrier of a faulty gene. Disorders inherited in such simple genetic fashion include sickle cell anemia and the thalassemias, phenylketonuria, Lesch-Nyhan disease, albinism, Tay-Sachs disease, cystic fibrosis, and hundreds of others. These are individually rare but collectively an enormous medical and social burden.

Monitoring for faulty genes in the preimplantation embryonic stage has the benefit of obviating anxiety stemming from diagnosis of the fetus *in utero* that involves invasive techniques such as amniocentesis. Prevention before implantation would circumvent the necessity of an abortion at a later stage of pregnancy. Even better, some thoughtful observers have argued, would be the replacement of the faulty gene with the normal gene so that the preimplantation embryo can be saved. Once proficiency is gained in monitoring genetic abnormalities in the embryo, is it inevitable that we will opt to correct the genetic defects in the embryo? This revolutionary kind of treatment known as *gene therapy* is the focal point of the concluding chapter of this book.

---

[17]Sickle cell anemia is associated with a gene that codes for a polypeptide chain (the *beta* chain) of the hemoglobin molecule. A particular restriction enzyme (designated Hpa I) recognizes the coding sequence in the DNA molecule that is responsible for the pattern of linked amino acids in the *beta* polypeptide chain. Three types of fragments bearing the gene that codes for the *beta* chain of hemoglobin are produced by digesting human DNA with the restriction enzyme Hpa I. The lengths of the fragments are delineated in kilobases (kb). The normal *beta* gene is located on a DNA fragment that is either 7.0 or 7.6 kb (7,000 or 7,600 nucleotides) in length. In contrast, the aberrant *beta* (sickle cell) gene is located on a fragment that is 13 kb long. This aberrant gene is associated with the loss of a recognition site for the restriction enzyme with the outcome that a larger than normal fragment (13 kb rather than 7.0 or 7.6 kb) is produced when the sickle cell DNA is cleaved. See Y. W. Kan and A. M. Dozy, "Antenatal Diagnosis of Sickle-Cell Anaemia by D.N.A. Analysis of Amniotic-Fluid Cells," *Lancet* 2 (1978): 910-12.

Chapter 6

Frozen Human Embryos

In most *in vitro* centers, fertility drugs are used to stimulate the woman to produce several preovulatory eggs. In American centers, physicians routinely transfer every fertilized egg into the woman's womb. Clinical experience has indicated, however, that the transfer of more than three embryos increases the chances of twins, triplets, and higher multiple births, with its attendant dangers to the mother and offspring. In recent years, Australian physicians have minimized obstetric risks associated with multiple pregnancies by implanting no more than three embryos at a time and freezing the remainder for future attempts. The spectacular technical success in the freezing (technically, cryopreservation) of embryos has become the subject of headlines and nationwide debate.

The first mammalian embryos to be successfully frozen and thawed were those of the mouse.[1] The preimplantation mouse embryo not only can survive temperatures as low as -196°C, but is able to develop into a normal offspring when transferred, after thawing, to a suitably prepared foster mother. Indeed, the mouse embryo can remain in storage for up to eight

---

[1] In 1972, two independent reports—one from Oak Ridge in the United States and the other from Cambridge University—described the first successful freezing of mouse embryos. See D. G. Whittingham, S. P. Leibo, and P. Masur, "Survival of Mouse Embryos Frozen to -196° and -269°C," *Science* 178 (1972): 411-14; I. Wilmut, "Effect of Cooling Rate, Warming Rate, Cryoprotective Agent and Stage of Development on Survival of Mouse Embryos during Cooling and Thawing," *Life Sciences* 11 (1972): 1071-79.

months (and possibly decades), and can even survive being transported in a small liquid nitrogen canister by air from one continent to another.[2] An even more remarkable finding is that ninety percent of frozen mouse embryos develop normally after thawing, and more than sixty-five percent of the frozen and thawed embryos transferred to the uterus yield viable offspring.[3] The procedures have now been perfected to include the embryos of several other mammalian species—rats, rabbits, sheep, goats, and cattle. The numerous trials thus far have revealed no evidence of major developmental abnormalities attributable to freezing and thawing. By this apparently safe technique, valuable strains of domestic animals can be protected against possible loss through disease or accident.[4]

The birth of the first baby to have been frozen as a test-tube embryo was announced in the Spring of 1984 by a team of Australian physicians at Monash University in Melbourne.[5] A normal baby girl (Zoe Leyland) was delivered after the successful transfer of two thawed embryos which had been frozen for eight weeks. The mother was a thirty-three-year old New Zealand woman who had been married for twelve years and had undergone two unsuccessful surgical operations to remove pelvic adhesions. In her first attempt at *in vitro* fertilization, eleven eggs were retrieved at laparoscopy and ten of these were inseminated with her husband's sperm. Three of the embryos were transferred to her uterus, but none resulted in pregnancy. Normally, Mrs. Leyland would have required another regimen of hormonal treatment and laparoscopy to obtain additional eggs. But she had earlier consented to the freezing of six embryos.[6] At the cou-

---

[2]D. G. Whittingham and W. K. Whitten, "Long-Term Storage and Aerial Transport of Frozen Mouse Embryos," *Journal of Reproduction and Fertility* 36 (1974): 433-35.

[3]Preliminary findings indicate that fifty to sixty percent of human embryos are viable after freezing and thawing. See J. Cohen, R. F. Simons, R. G. Edwards, C. B. Fehilly, and S. B. Fishel, "Pregnancies Following the Frozen Storage of Expanding Human Blastocysts," *Journal of In Vitro Fertilization and Embryo Transfer* 2 (1985): 59-66; L. R. Mohr, A. Trounson, L. Freeman, "Deep Freezing and Transfer of Human Embryos," *Journal of In Vitro Fertilization and Embryo Transfer* 2 (1985): 1-9.

[4]Ciba Foundation, *The Freezing of Mammalian Embryos,* Ciba Foundation Symposium 52, new series (London: Elsevier, 1977).

[5]B. C. Downing, L. R. Mohr, L. E. Freeman, A. O. Trounson et al. "Birth After Transfer of Cryopreserved Embryos," *Medical Journal of Australia* 142 (1985): 409-11.

[6]To date, pregnancies can be achieved after freezing and thawing of eight-cell human

ple's request, the frozen embryos were thawed after two months in storage and two embryos were transferred to her uterus. On that second occasion, a pregnancy progressed normally.

The foregoing case history vividly illustrates the new dimensions afforded by the freeze-thaw procedure. The freezing of the unused embryos provides parents with a new option: a second attempt at implantation at a subsequent occasion if the first attempt is unsuccessful. Indeed, there may be successive pregnancies several years later. The new option entails only one surgical procedure, avoiding the discomfort and cost of repeated laparoscopies to recover eggs. Additionally, the combination of superovulation and freeze preservation allows for deliberately delaying embryo transfer until a more suitable occasion when the uterus has been prepared by the woman's own spontaneous hormonal cycle. The chances of successful implantation of the embryo are likely to be higher by relying on the woman's undisturbed hormonal pattern.[7]

The Australian physicians regard the freezing of human embryos as a logical extension of earlier work to ensure a higher success rate of pregnancy. Several normal infants (including one pair of twins) have now been born in Melbourne after freezing and thawing, and at least two have been delivered in the Netherlands.[8] A clinic at the Good Samaritan Hospital in Los Angeles, headed by Dr. Richard Mars, has adapted the freeze-thaw protocol of the Australian workers. In early June 1986, Dr. Mars an-

---

embryos cooled at 0.3°C per minute to $-80°C$ in the presence of 1.5 molar dimethyl sulfoxide (DMSO) and thawed at $+8°C$ per minute from $-80°C$ to $+4°C$. By this procedure, more than fifty percent of the embryos survive without any developmental abnormalities. See L. R. Mohr and A. O. Trounson, "Cryopreservation of Human Embryos," *Annals New York Academy of Science* 442 (1985): 536-43.

[7]Women whose ovulatory cycles have been stimulated with clomiphene citrate and gonadotropins may experience a diminished capacity for implantation, which probably reflects an inadequate uterine response associated with a reduced length of the luteal phase. See J. J. Cohen, C. Debache, F. Pigeau, J. Mandelbaum, et al., "Sequential Use of Clomiphene Citrate, Human Menopausal Gonadotropin, and Human Chorionic Gonadotropin in Human *in Vitro* Fertilization. II. Study of Luteal Phase Adequacy Following Aspiration of the Preovulatory Follicles," *Fertility and Sterility* 42 (1984): 360-65.

[8]G. H. Zeilmaker, A. Th. Aberda, I. Van Gent, C. M. P. M. Rijkamans et al., "Two Pregnancies Following Transfer of Intact Frozen-Thawed Embryos," *Fertility and Sterility* 42 (1984): 293-96.

nounced that a normal nine-pound, ten-ounce boy had been delivered to an American woman who had been implanted with a thawed embryo.[9]

In spite of the inescapable advantages, the freezing of the live human embryos spurs issues that go beyond those raised by *in vitro* fertilization in general. The thorny issues were punctuated by an event in the spring of 1984 that was so bizarre that it could have been written by an imaginative novelist.[10] An American couple from Los Angeles, Mario and Elsa Rios perished in a plane crash, leaving behind two frozen embryos at the Queen Victoria Medical Center in Melbourne, Australia. Earlier, at the Melbourne Medical Center, three preovulatory eggs had been removed from Mrs. Rios and successfully fertilized *in vitro*. One of the embryos was implanted in her uterus; the other two were frozen for possible use in the future. Mrs. Rios subsequently miscarried, but she was not emotionally prepared at that time to undertake further implantations with the frozen embryos. With her death, what are the rights of the frozen embryos? Do these embryos have a right to life through implantation in a surrogate mother? The situation is even more dramatic in that the parents died intestate (without a will) with a substantial inheritance at stake. And there is now the admission that the deceased husband was not the father of the embryos; rather, the sperm was contributed by an anonymous donor in Melbourne.[11]

The act of placing an embryo in storage serves to prolong the embryo's existence outside the mother's body. The longer the event of storage, the greater the autonomy of the embryo. Whereas an embryo remains in developmental stasis in its frozen state, the mother ages with time and uterine receptivity declines. How does the passage of time affect the status of the embryo? In other words, to whom does a frozen embryo belong? For the first time, the human embryo has been endowed with a unique capabil-

---

[9]"First in U.S.: Healthy Boy Is Born After Frozen Embryo Implantation," *The Atlanta Journal*, 5 June 1986, 9A.

[10]D. T. Ozar, "The Case against Thawing Unused Frozen Embryos," *Hastings Center Report* 15 (1985): 7-12; G. P. Smith II, "Australia's Frozen 'Orphan' Embryos: A Medical, Legal, and Ethical Dilemma," *Journal of Family Law* 24 (1985-86): 27-41.

[11]In October 1984, legislators in the state of Victoria rejected a recommendation of a committee that the two frozen embryos, left in legal limbo by the death of their mother and her husband, be destroyed (*New York Times,* 24 October 1984). Victoria's Parliament passed an amendment to a bill, calling for an attempt to have the two embryos implanted in a surrogate mother and then placed for adoption.

ity—the capacity to mature into an individual completely independent of its genetic parents, both physically and in time.[12]

American scientists are keenly aware of the need for ethical as well as technical guidelines in dealing with the complex issue of frozen embryos. In the United States, in the absence of federal support of *in vitro* fertilization research, there are no government decisions or policies on any of the novel reproductive options. The hope, however, is that guidelines or criteria for clinics will emerge from the medical community rather than from legal restrictions. One able spokesman for the scientific community has been Clifford Grobstein at the University of California in San Diego.[13] He advocates that the storage time for frozen embryos be limited to that required for its initial purpose—namely, a subsequent pregnancy to the same couple. The embryo should be stored for a maximum period equivalent to the natural reproductive capabilities of the individual woman—until menopause or until such time that the couple should no longer live together. The American Fertility Society underscores that a transfer of embryos from one generation to another is wholly unacceptable.[14]

George Annas, Professor of Health Law at the Boston University School of Medicine tends to agree that the federal government should stay out of the arena of human reproduction. But he has expressed concern that frozen embryos might be used for purposes other that their specified purpose.[15] He has urged the establishment of a national body of experts in law, public policy, science, medicine, and ethics to monitor developments in reproductive technology and report to Congress on the desirability of specific regulation and legislation. Such national committees exist in Britain and Australia, which have published recommendations that are intended as standards for clinics involved in *in vitro* fertilization, including embryo

---

[12]The freezing of the egg in the unfertilized state might raise fewer ethical and legal questions than the storage of embryos. However, although the ability to freeze and store human sperm cells is a well-established procedure, success has yet to be achieved for the safe storage of an unfertilized egg (oocyte).

[13]C. M. Grobstein, M. Flower, and J. Mendeloff, "Frozen embryos: Policy issues," *New England Journal of Medicine* 312 (1985): 1584-88.

[14]Ethics Committee of the American Fertility Society, "Ethical Considerations of the New Reproductive Technologies," *Fertility and Sterility* 46, Supplement 1 (1986): 1-94.

[15]G. J. Annas, "Redefining Parenthood and Protecting Embryos: Why We Need New Laws," *The Hastings Center Report* 14 (1984): 50-52

freezing. On the basis of committee recommendations, the Victoria Parliament in Australia has become the first jurisdiction in the world to enact comprehensive legislation that sets firm limits on the new reproductive technologies.[16]

The Infertility Act, passed by the Victoria Parliament in the first week of November 1984, specifies that all patients must have been under treatment for infertility for at least one year before *in vitro* fertilization is attempted. This provision is intended to ensure that the *in vitro* treatment is clearly one of "last resort" for infertile couples. The new law permits the freezing of embryos, only to the extent that the freeze-thaw procedure is carried out with the aim of implanting the embryo in the womb of a woman at a later date. Finally, the new law prohibits any kind of commercial market in human reproductive material—that is, no payment may be made for sperm, egg, or embryo. Since there is almost universal consensus that human kidneys should not be bought or sold, it would seem that society would also wish to protect the human embryo from commercial exploitation.

---

[16]P. Singer, "Making Laws on Making Babies," *Hastings Center Report* 15 (1985): 5-6.

Chapter 7

Surrogate Mothers

A surrogate mother is a substitute performer, one who takes the place of another woman. She is a person who, for financial or compassionate reasons, carries the child of another woman with the intent of surrendering the child to that woman.[1] As applicable to *in vitro* fertilization, the egg and sperm come from the commissioning couple, but the resulting embryo is implanted in a woman who agrees to act as a surrogate mother. Thus, the child belongs biologically to the contracting couple, and the proxy gestational mother who, though having carried the child, has no genetic ties to the child. The surrogate performs the unusual service for a substantial fee, and relinquishes all rights to the child at birth.[2] In the United States alone,

---

[1]Surrogacy is not a new concept; the practice was condoned in the Old Testament. It was acceptable for a woman other than the wife to bear the couple's child, as in the case of Rachel, denied of motherhood, having her slave-girl bear a child with her husband Jacob (Genesis 13) or as witnessed by Abram's wife Sarai asking her husband Abram to obtain a child for her through her maid-servant Hagar (Genesis 16, Revised Standard Version).

[2]Prior to the advent of *in vitro* fertilization, surrogate motherhood had a different dimension. Either the husband of the commissioning couple impregnated the surrogate by the sexual act, or the impregnation occurred by artificial insemination. Accordingly, the child was only partially related biologically to the couple. The modern form of surrogacy that makes use of *in vitro* fertilization has been characterized as "rent-a-womb" surrogacy by imaginative journalists. Since the surrogate mother provides the gestational component but not the genetic ingredient, some writers prefer the very explicit expression "surrogate gestational mother."

it is estimated that several hundred women are currently, or have been, fulfilling roles as surrogate mothers.[3]

There are certain circumstances in which surrogacy would seem to be a reasonable option. Some women are medically incapable of either becoming pregnant or carrying a fetus to term, whether by normal means or by *in vitro* fertilization. Some of the more serious medical impairments that drastically curtail a woman's reproductive capacity are life-threatening kidney disorders, severe diabetes, debilitating cardiac disease, and a history of repeated miscarriages. For many of these women, adoption is no longer a viable alternative because of the diminishing numbers of babies available for adoption and the generally long waiting period associated with the adoption procedure. More importantly, surrogacy offers the only chance of having a child that has a genetic link to the couple. In this respect, surrogacy is a better alternative to adoption. It is natural for couples to prefer genetically related children over biologically unrelated children.

Surrogacy is technologically feasible, but is it morally defensible? Some ethicists object to surrogacy on the grounds that the practice constitutes economic exploitation of women. The carrying of a child is traditionally an intimate affair, and it should be an affront to one's moral and aesthetic sensibility that such an event is blatantly commercialized. Detractors point out that it is as morally distasteful for a woman to bear a child for money as it is for a woman to ask money for sexual favors. Scientists themselves acknowledge that surrogacy is not a new medical advance but rather a commercial enterprise wherein motherhood is determined by contract. The only "new" development is the hiring of attorneys who, for a fee, recruit women who are willing, for a price, to allow themselves to be used as human incubators and are willing to relinquish their gestational rights to the child. The novelty thus lies in treating babies like commodities.[4] The myr-

---

[3]In the United States, the first pregnancy of a surrogate gestational mother was reported in 1985 by clinicians at the Mt. Sinai Medical Center in Cleveland, Ohio; a successful birth ensued in April 1986. See U. H. Utian, L. Sheehan, J. M. Goldfarb, and R. Kiwi, "Successful Pregnancy After in Vitro Fertilization and Embryo Transfer from an Infertile Woman to a Surrogate," *New England Journal of Medicine* 313 (1985): 1351-52; P. Chargot and B. Flanigan, "First Baby Born by Surrogate via Test Tube," *Detroit Free Press,* 17 April 1986, 1A.

[4]Noel Deane, an enterprising Michigan lawyer who arranges contracts between infertile couples and surrogate women, has written of his experiences in a revealing book entitled *The Surrogate Mother* (New York: Everest House, 1981). Typically, the commissioning

iad problems of surrogacy are underscored by the pithy query in the *New York Times* (31 July 1978), "Which One Gets the Mother's Day Card?"

What would motivate a woman to place herself in the role of a surrogate mother? A priori one might presume that the applicants are desperate women who are unemployed or on welfare roles. On the contrary, the available data reveal that the decision to be a surrogate springs from motives other than pecuniary.[5] Most surrogates have been in the mid-twenties, married, religious (mainly Catholics and Protestants), with formal education ranging from less than high school to the bachelor's degree. The surrogates viewed themselves as bestowing the gift of life to another couple. They immensely enjoyed the state of pregnancy, as a truly creative experience. The group as a whole felt content and special during pregnancy, and enjoyed the extra attention bestowed upon them. Surrogacy has helped some women resolve unhappy feelings from past pregnancies that ended electively in abortion or adoption. But the emotional toll of delivery is great. On relinquishing the child to the contracting couple, the surrogate experiences feelings of loss, depression, and guilt. In several instances, surrogate mothers have fought to keep the children they bore.[6] It should be apparent that surrogate motherhood is not at all comparable to AID (artificial insemination by donor), since the contribution of the gestational mother is greater, more intimate and personal, than the investment of a sperm donor. The difference in physical and emotional investment is tacitly acknowledged in economic terms: the compensation is $100 or less for the sperm donor as compared to $10,000 for the surrogate mother.

Whatever the motives, the surrogate mother is certainly more than a passive incubator. A variety of substances—nutrients, waste products, antibodies, viruses, and drugs—find their way across the placenta from the mother to the developing fetus. The fetus is not protected from such harmful chemical or physical agents as sleeping pills (thalidomide), tranquil-

---

couple will need at least $22,000: $10,000 for the surrogate mother's fee, $5,000 for medical expenses, $5,000 for legal fees to draw up the contract and arrange the eventual adoption of the baby, and about $2,000 for miscellaneous expenses. There are surrogate mother centers in Michigan, Kentucky, California, Maryland, Arizona, and several other states. There is even a surrogate mother newsletter.

[5]P. J. Parker, "Motivation of Surrogate Mothers: Initial Findings," *American Journal of Psychiatry* 40 (1983): 117-18.

[6]L. B. Andrews, "The Stork Market: The Law of the New Reproduction Technologies," *American Bar Association Journal* 70 (1984): 50-56.

izers (meprobromate), barbituates (sodium barbital), and certain antibiotics (streptomycin).[7] Maternal diseases such as diabetes, syphilis, tuberculosis, and German measles also represent potential danger to the developing fetus. Improper diet, excessive smoking, and alcohol may also interfere with proper development or delivery of the fetus. Given these circumstances, may the couple place restrictions on the habits, the medical care, or the diet of the surrogate? Can the surrogate, for example, be limited to a certain weekly intake of alcohol or be prohibited from smoking? It is highly unlikely that a court of law would order a surrogate to perform services of a very personal nature.[8]

The vast problems, potential and actual, appear almost insurmountable. If complications in the pregnancy occur, then profound questions are raised for which no firm solutions are available. Could the surrogate be made to undergo amniocentesis, so as to monitor fetal abnormalities? Could the couple require that the surrogate undergo an abortion if there is unequivocal evidence of fetal deformity? What if a malformed child is born? These considerations are not purely hypothetical. In 1977, a Michigan couple arranged a surrogate contract with a woman living in Tennessee, who seemed to be a responsible person. The woman, however, was an alcoholic, and in 1978 she gave birth to a child with a condition now recognized medically as "fetal alcohol syndrome." Aside from suffering from drug-withdrawal symptoms, the newborn infant had below normal weight and height and a prognosis, in later life, of impairment of mental ability. In another touching case, a Michigan surrogate mother, in January 1983, gave birth to a child with microcephaly, a condition in which the head is abnormally small with attendant mental retardation.[9] Even if all parties concerned were to specify the liabilities in a contract, there is no assurance that the specifications would be judicially recognized or enforced.

---

[7]E. P. Volpe, *Patient in the Womb* (Macon GA: Mercer University Press, 1984) 123-29.

[8]S. Taub, "Surrogate Motherhood and the Law," *Connecticut Medicine* 49 (1985): 671-74.

[9]Neither the contracting couple nor the surrogate mother wanted to accept the microcephalic infant. Ironically, it turned out that the surrogate had actually borne her husband's child, as she had unwittingly become pregnant by him prior to the contractual arrangement with the infertile couple. The surrogate and her husband finally accepted responsibility for the child (*New York Times,* 28 January 1983, 18).

It is almost unfathomable how a judge would resolve a dispute between the child's genetic mother and the child's gestational surrogate mother. If a surrogate desires to breach the contract by abortion and the judge were to order her to continue the pregnancy, it would be difficult to enforce or monitor the order. If the surrogate declined to relinquish the child after birth, the Court would have to decide whether the child's interest would best be served by the surrogate or the genetic parents. The genetic parents would more often than not be favored since the greatest yardstick would be the biological input.[10] Yet, there is likely to be sympathy for the gestational bond between the surrogate mother and child.

In the Summer of 1986, a County Superior Court in New Jersey began hearings on a celebrated case in which a surrogate mother was unwilling to give up the baby after birth.[11] Mrs. Mary Beth Whitehead in 1985 consented to artificial insemination using sperm from William Stern, a forty-year-old biochemist residing in New Jersey. His wife, Elizabeth, a forty-year-old pediatrician, agreed to pay $10,000 to Mrs. Whitehead on the condition that the latter relinquish all rights to the baby at birth. Elizabeth Stern resorted to a surrogate arrangement because she suffered from multiple sclerosis, an unquestionable health risk in pregnancy. After the birth of the child, Mrs. Whitehead claimed she was too emotionally attached to the infant to give it up. A state judge ruled that the Sterns could retain custody of the infant girl until a final ruling by a higher court. The Superior Court was now confronted with the necessity of resolving a novel problem for which there are no legal precedents or guidance.[12] It was anticipated that the case would be treated solely as a contract dispute and that the judge's decision would not be based on deep ethical reflections. Indeed, on 31

---

[10]D. J. Cusine, "Some Legal Implications of Embryo Transfer?", *New Law Journal* 28 (1979): 627-28.

[11]"In Court Battle for Baby M, Emotions are Fierce," *New York Times,* 23 August 1986, 8; "Father Recalls Surrogate was 'Perfect'," *New York Times,* 6 January 1987, 15; "Baby M, Ethics and the Law," *New York Times,* 18 January 1987, 1; "Father of Baby M Granted Custody; Contract Upheld," *New York Times,* 1 April 1987, 1.

[12]The presiding judge might covet the wisdom of King Solomon to decide the fate of the child and its parents. When confronted by two women claiming the same child, King Solomon ordered that the child be split in two and one half given to each mother. The true mother, not wishing to see her child destroyed, chose to give up the child to the other woman. Upon witnessing her great love for the child, King Solomon was able to determine the true parent, and thus awarded the child to her (1 Kings 3:16-28).

March, 1987 the judge denied the surrogate mother any parental rights and upheld the $10,000 contract under which she agreed to give up the child.

The numerous legal questions are bewildering and remain largely unresolved. Some states, like Michigan and Kentucky, have attempted to disallow surrogacy contractual arrangements on the grounds that the contracts violate historical criminal statutes that prohibit "baby selling." However, the original statutes against the sale of a child were intended to protect women from being coerced into selling their children. The surrogate mother does not enter into a contractual agreement under coercion, and it is unlikely that any form of criminal prohibition of surrogate motherhood can be enforced. Indeed, in 1986, the Supreme Court of Kentucky declared that surrogate motherhood does not violate the state's prohibition against the purchase of any child for the purpose of adoption. The Court ruled that the fee paid to the surrogate mother is for her services, which include the physical acts of pregnancy and childbirth, and not for the child itself.

Opposition to surrogate motherhood is widespread. Over the past few years, several committees, in the United States and abroad, have published guidelines on various aspects of the new reproductive technologies. In 1982, a committee in England was established under Dame Mary Warnock, with its sixteen members representing scientific, religious, legal, and lay viewpoints. The long-awaited Warnock report, published in 1984, summarily rejected surrogacy arrangements.[13] In fact, the committee recommended that legislation be introduced to render criminal the creation or the operation in the United Kingdom of agencies offering surrogacy services. Two members of the committee dissented, maintaining that there were occasions when surrogacy could be salutary to couples "as a last resort."

The argument for criminal prosecution is unimpressive to some authors.[14] Any new law to prohibit surrogacy agreements would probably be futile, if only because prohibition would encourage underground trade. Instead, lawmakers would do better to focus on constructive methods of *regulating* the practice. The regulations would be concerned with delineating

---

[13]*Report of the Committee of Enquiry into Human Fertilization and Embryology,* Department of Health and Social Security, Her Majesty's Stationery Office, London, 1984.

[14]J. A. Robertson, "Surrogate Mothers: Not So Novel at All," *The Hastings Center Report* 13 (1983): 28-34.

the varied precautions to be observed, particularly the level of medical fitness of the surrogate mother. For example, the Courts could set minimum standards for the age and health qualifications of the surrogates. The government or state could also define the conditions that protect the best interests of the offspring. The law could also set a maximum fee for the service. In essence, careful and detailed legislative regulation is needed to promote the interests of all parties. A cardinal question is whether access to the services of a surrogate should be restricted soley to those people who, for medical reasons, are unable to bear a child. Should the services be denied to those women who, though physically capable of giving birth, do not do so either because they are too busy or because their careers are too demanding? Are such reasons too frivolous or misplaced?

Chapter 8

Expanding Horizons

Medical researchers continue unabated in their search for new approaches in the treatment of infertility. One novel procedure that has considerable promise has been called GIFT, an acronym for "Gamete Intra-Fallopian Transfer." The GIFT procedure was developed at the University of Texas Health Science Center at San Antonio by a research team headed by Dr. Richardo Asch.[1] The procedure basically imitates the normal sequence of fertilization events by bringing the egg and sperm together in the woman's fallopian tubes (figure 14). About sixty-five percent of infertile couples can be helped by this procedure. The treatment is particularly suited to those couples with problems of unexplained infertility or where the female partner has a cervix that does not permit sperm penetration. It is also a clinical option in those cases where the male partner has inadequate sperm. The GIFT procedure is not helpful to women with blocked fallopian tubes.

The advantage of GIFT compared to *in vitro* fertilization is that the fertilized egg is allowed to develop in its passage through the fallopian tube rather than in laboratory glassware—a close parallel to what occurs naturally. Additionally, fewer steps are involved; the eggs are removed and implanted in the same procedure rather than removed one day and transferred several days later as in *in vitro* fertilization. As with conventional

---

[1]R. H. Asch, J. P. Balmaceda, L. R. Ellsworth, and P. C. Wong, "Gamete Intra-Fallopian Transfer (GIFT): A New Treatment for Infertility," *International Journal of Fertility* 30 (1985): 41-45.

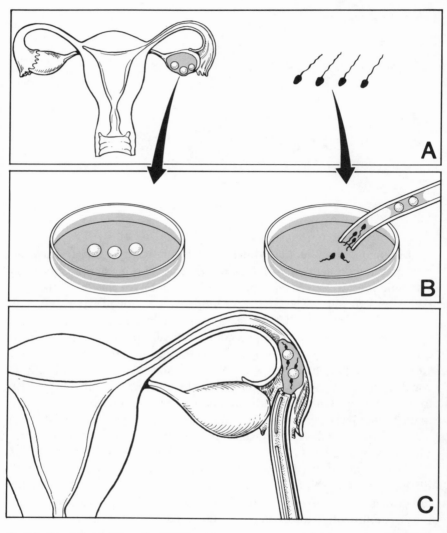

Gamete Intrafallopian Transfer (GIFT)

Figure 14

Eggs and sperm are placed in separate culture dishes (A), and then transferred unmixed via a catheter (B) into the fallopian tube where fertilization takes place (C).

in vitro fertilization, the woman is induced by hormones to produce several eggs, which are aspirated by laparoscopy. The husband's semen sample had been obtained two hours earlier. The eggs and sperm preparation are placed in a catheter, but an intentionally created air space separates the gametes and precludes their contact or mixture. The loaded catheter is then inserted into the woman's fallopian tube through the same laparoscope used for aspirating the eggs. Fertilization thus takes place in the fallopian tube, and the embryo descends into the uterus in the normal manner. Since there is no contact of gametes *in vivo* nor any possibility of embryo manipulation, the GIFT technique may be ethically acceptable to a larger segment of society. About 300 GIFT pregnancies have been achieved in the United States and abroad since the inception of the technique in 1984.

There is a relatively small, but not unimportant, group of young women who in the past had scarcely any hope whatever of conceiving a child. These women either lack ovaries or have nonfunctional ovaries.[2] Such a woman cannot have a child that is genetically her own, but she can now realistically consider receiving an egg from a fertile woman that has been fertilized by the sperm of her husband. This new variation on the theme is known as "nonsurgical ovum transfer," "embryo donation by uterine flushing," and colloquially as "intrauterine adoption." The procedure involves the artificial insemination of an egg of a fertile donor with the semen of a man whose wife is infertile. Before the fertilized egg has the opportunity to implant in the donor's uterus, it is removed and transferred to the infertile wife's uterus. The infertile wife carries the embryo to term.[3] The technique came into prominence after Dr. Gary Hodgen at the National Institutes of Health demonstrated in 1983 the feasibility of establishing a normal pregnancy in rhesus monkeys even in the complete absence of ovarian

---

[2]In women with an inherited condition called "gonadal dysgenesis," the ovaries are absent or are replaced by a whitish streak of fibrous tissue. Gonadal dysgenesis characteristically occurs in women who are missing one X chromosome (45, XO). There are also chromosomally normal women who experience "premature ovarian failure." In the majority of these women, the ovaries atrophy and become completely devoid of egg follicles before the age of thirty-five.

[3]The nonsurgical transfer of a fertilized egg from donor to recipient was successfully undertaken in mice by Beatty in 1951. The technique is now extensively used in cattle breeding. See R. A. Beatty, "Transplantation of Mouse Eggs," *Nature* 168 (1951): 995; G. E. Seidel, Jr., "Superovulation and embryo transfer in cattle," *Science* 211 (1981): 351-58.

function.[4] Hodgen showed that, in a monkey without ovaries, proper doses of estrogen and progesterone alone can provide a suitable hormonal environment for a successful pregnancy.

The findings by Hodgen encouraged clinical investigations in humans using embryo donation in conjunction with hormonal replacement therapy in women lacking ovarian function. Reports of success in humans soon followed. In July 1983, two pregnancies by embryo donation were announced by Dr. Marian Bustillo and her colleagues at the Harbor-UCLA Medical Center in Torrance, California.[5] The donor women were between the ages of twenty-six and thirty-five years. Psychological screening test revealed that they were free of major emotional problems. The recipients were married women between the ages of twenty-three and thirty-six years. In each case, the fertile donor woman and the husband of the infertile couple agreed to abstain sexually during the preovulatory period—namely, five days prior to the anticipated luteinizing hormone (LH) peak. Insemination of the donor woman with semen from the infertile recipient's husband was perfomed on the day of the LH peak, the predicted time of ovulation. Fertilization was thus allowed to occur in the reproductive tract of the donor woman. From five to seven days after the donor's LH peak, continual attempts were made to recover the fertilized egg by flushing the uterine cavity of the donor, a procedure known as *lavage*. Once an embryo was recovered, the lavage sequence was terminated. The lavage fluid was scanned in a flat culture dish to recover the embryo. The embryo was transferred to the infertile recipient woman.

There is presently limited experience with this reproductive technology. At the Harbor-UCLA Medical Center, there have been three intrauterine pregnancies and one ectopic pregnancy.[6] Normal term infants resulted from two of the intrauterine pregnancies; the third pregnancy re-

---

[4]G. D. Hodgen, "Surrogate embryo transfer combined with estrogen-progesterone therapy in monkeys," *Journal of the American Medical Association* 250 (1983): 2167-71.

[5]M. Bustillo, J. E. Buster, S. W. Cohen, I. H. Thorneycroft, et al., "Nonsurgical Ovum Transfer as a Treatment in Infertile Women," *Journal of the American Medical Association* 251 (1984): 1171-73.

[6]J. E. Buster, M. Bustillo, I. A. Rodi, S. W. Cohen, et al., *Biologic and Morphologic Development of Donated Human Ova Recovered by Nonsurgical Uterine Lavage,"* American Journal of Obstetrics and Gynecology* 153 (1985): 211-17; J. E. Buster, "Embryo Donation by Uterine Flushing and Embryo Transfer," ed. C. Wood and A. Trounson. *Clinics in Obstetrics and Gynecology* 12 (London: W. B. Saunders Co., 1985) 815-24.

sulted in a spontaneous abortion at thirteen weeks. The ectopic pregnancy was terminated surgically. Despite all the vicissitudes, embryo donation by uterine flushing has become a viable clinical option. A grave circumstance can arise if a uterine pregnancy inadvertently ensues in the donor woman because the lavage procedure fails to retrieve the embryo from the donor's uterine cavity. The embryo donor would then confront a decision about the continuation of a unexpected pregnancy. From a strictly scientific viewpoint, an important thesis has been validated: even though a woman lacks ovaries, her uterus can be prepared to receive an embryo by the administration of estrogen and progesterone. Confirmation of the establishment of pregnancies in the absence of ovaries has now come from different parts of the world—Australia[7] in 1984 and Israel[8] in 1986.

The process of donating an embryo, although more complicated, is analogous to artificial insemination by donor (AID) in that the genetic contribution comes from one parent only. In fact, intrauterine adoption might raise fewer problems for the marriage relation than AID because both husband and wife each makes a contribution: the husband contributes the sperm and the wife provides the entire uterine environment throughout pregnancy, enhancing the mother-child bond. As compared to other medical practices, both AID and intrauterine adoption are so confidential, or secret, that anonymity of the donor is considered a virtue. The confidentiality obliges the physician, the husband and wife, and the donor to conspire together to deceive the child as to its true parentage—its genetic identity. It is commonly assumed that it is in the child's best interest that he or she be so deceived. This assumption may or may not be warranted. We have insufficient data to judge whether a child's psychological needs would be seriously harmed by the truth, or at what age he or she might safely learn of his or her true parentage.[9] For many children, the strong psychological

---

[7]P. Lutjen, A. Trounson, J. Leeton, J. Findlay, et al., "The Establishment and Maintenance of Pregnancy Using *in Vitro* Fertilization and Embryo Donation in a Patient with Primary Ovarian Failure." *Nature* 307 (1984): 174-75.

[8]D. Navot, N. Laufer, J. Kopolovic, R. Rabinowitz, et al., "Artificially induced endometrial cycles and establishment of pregnancies in the absence of ovaries," *New England Journal of Medicine* 314 (1986): 806-11.

[9]A strong justification for secrecy is to protect the sperm donor from any claims that the child may make. See A. D. Sorosky, A. Bavan, and R. Pannor. *The Adoption Triangle.* (Garden City: Anchor Press, 1978); M. Curie-Cohen, L. Luttrell, and S. Shapiro, "Current Practice of Artificial Insemination by Donor in the United States," *New England Journal of Medicine* 300 (1979): 588-90.

need to know one's biological parents favors disclosure.[10] The parental attitude toward the child is important; any sense of guilt on the part of the
parents because they have refrained from telling the truth would certainly
affect the child's self-image. At issue also is the integrity of the medical
profession. It is a matter of serious concern that the medical community,
which places such a high value on truth, should in fact promote, if not require, purposeful deception.

---

[10]The principal argument against disclosure is that the donor wants his or her identity
to be kept confidential. In 1984, Sweden passed legislation that gives a child conceived by
A.I.D., upon reaching 18 years of age, the right to learn of the identity of the genetic father.
During the relatively short period of time that the law has been in effect, donor insemination has declined precipitously as if to suggest that donors seek neither recognition nor responsibility.

Chapter 9

Sex Selection

Ideally, most parents desire both sons and daughters, a goal that was nearly always achieved when large families were customary. However, with the contemporary Western imperative on limiting family size, the sex composition of the children figures prominently in the planning of smaller families. Studies by sociologists reveal that the maternal preference for sons is pervasive in the American culture.[1] Most women want a two-child family with a strong desire that the firstborn be a son.[2] If many parents were to satisfy their partiality for firstborn sons, the impact on daughters might be unfavorable. What are the implications of being second-born as well as second choice? Although experts have forecast profound social, psychological, and demographic consequences of sex selection, there is no unanimity on what exactly these consequences would be. Nevertheless, the technology that permits couples to choose the sex of their children is rap-

[1]L. C. Coombs, "Preferences for Sex of Children among U.S. Couples," *Family Planning Perspectives* 9 (1977): 259-65; N. E. Williamson, "Boys or girls? Parents' Preferences and Sex Control" *Population Bulletin* 33 (Washington: Population Reference Bureau, 1978).

[2]The three reasons most often stated by women for desiring sons as firstborn were (1) to please their husbands, (2) to carry on the family name, and (3) to provide a companion for the husband. See A. R. Pebley and C. F. Westhoff, "Women's Sex Preferences in the United States: 1970 to 1975," *Demography* 19 (1982): 177-89.

idly being refined.[3] Is the use of such improved technology defensible, particularly if the number of couples having only one child increases?

There are two general strategies for predetermining, prior to conception, the sex of the unborn child. The first approach is based on the timing of intercourse in relation to ovulation. The second scheme involves the processing of the semen to separate the X-bearing and Y-bearing sperm, followed by artificial insemination of the woman with the fraction appropriate to the sex of the offspring desired. It is the chromosomal type of sperm that prescribes the genetic basis for maleness or femaleness. The sperm cell contains either an X or Y chromosome; only the X chromosome resides in the egg cell. The union of an X-bearing sperm with the egg produces a female (XX), while fertilization by a Y-bearing sperm results in a male (XY).

There are a far greater number of male conceptions, for reasons that are largely unknown.[4] It seems likely that equal numbers of X-bearing and Y-bearing sperm are produced, although the possibility of unequal production in favor of Y-bearing sperm cannot be discounted. It has been suggested that the Y-bearing sperm is more viable than the X-bearing sperm, or more proficient in fertilization. It has also been hypothesized that the Y-bearing sperm has a greater chance of reaching and penetrating the egg. The X chromosome is larger than the Y chromosome, and accordingly has a greater mass. Since velocity is influenced by mass, the sperm carrying

---

[3]The idea of exercising control over the sex of one's offspring is as old as recorded medical history. The ancient Hebrews believed that each testicle harbored semen of one sex: the right testicle contained male semen, while the left testicle contained female semen. The male needed only to tie off the appropriate testicle to obtain the desired sex. The practice persisted as late as the 1700s in Europe, where French noblemen who desired a male heir were advised to have their left testicle surgically removed. The Hebrew Talmud proclaimed that sex was determined by the direction of the wind at the time of coition. The conception of boys was favored if the marriage bed was placed on a north-south axis. See C. Zirkle, "The Knowledge of Heredity Before 1900," in L. C. Dunn, ed., *Genetics and the 20th Century* (New York: Macmillan and Co.; 1958) 35-55.

[4]Despite a twelve percent higher mortality rate of males *in utero*, approximately 106 boys are born for every 100 girls. The mortality rate among males is higher at all ages, and is evidenced in the first days of life. Females enjoy a thirty-two percent lower mortality rate in the first week of life and are less subject to sudden infant death. The male-to-female ratio drops to 100:100 at age twenty, and progressively declines therafter to reach the staggering figure of sixty-two males for every 100 females at age eighty-five. There are no satisfactory explanations for the higher male mortality. Part of the higher male mortality may be attributable to X-linked detrimental genes. (It has been mockingly stated that being a male became hazardous ever since Adam lost a rib.)

the Y chromosome should be able to travel in the female reproductive tract at a greater speed with the same amount of energy than the sperm bearing the X chromosome. This assumed ability became the basis of one of the more popular theories of sex preselection, promulgated by Dr. Landrum Shettles of the Columbia University College of Physicians and Surgeons.

In 1961, Shettles popularized the notion that a male offspring is more likely to be conceived from intercourse close to the time of ovulation.[5] According to Shettles, the Y-bearing sperm not only moves more rapidly in the female reproductive canal than the X-bearing sperm, but loses fertilizing capability more quickly. Therefore, if insemination occurs shortly after ovulation (when the egg is in the upper reaches of the fallopian tube), the Y-bearing sperm is more likely to reach the egg first. Conversely, if insemination takes place several days before ovulation, most Y-bearing sperm will be nonviable before the egg becomes available for fertilization.

Other strategies recommended by Shettles have captured the public imagination. Presumably the sex of the offspring could be controlled by adjusting the acidity or alkalinity of the fluids in the vagina. An alkaline condition, such as that brought about by the introduction of sodium bicarbonate into the vagina, was judged to increase the rate of migration of Y-bearing sperm, and accordingly, to increase the proportion of male conceptions. Conversely, an acid douche (2 tablespoons of white vinegar to 1 quart of water) would favor a female child. Although some publicity-gaining claims have been made, careful investigations have failed to provide supporting evidence.[6] Nor is there any evidence to support the contention that the sex of the offspring may be influenced by the presence or absence of female orgasm and the position or degree of male penetration at intercourse.

Shettles had hoped to derive support for his assertions from the higher ratio of male to female births arising from artificial insemination with donor sperm (AID). Since AID is performed as close as possible to the moment of ovulation, this would seem to indicate that the conception of a male child is associated with the closeness of ovulation. But the scientific com-

---

[5]L. B. Shettles, "Conception and Birth Sex Ratios: A Review," *Obstetrics and Gynecology* 18 (1961): 122-30.

[6]K. H. Broer, I. Winkhaus, H. Sombroek, and R. Kaiser, "Frequency of Y-Chromatin-Bearing Spermatozoa in Intracervical and Intrauterine Postcoital Tests," *International Journal of Fertility* 21 (1976): 181-86.

munity and the public were soon to be confounded by a study in 1974 by Dr. R. Guerrero that showed that artificial insemination provides an effect opposite that of normal intercourse.[7] Guerrero's investigation, as well as more recent studies,[8] indicate that the sex ratio favors males, the *longer* the interval between intercourse and ovulation.

Against this background of strategies that have been found wanting, it was not surprising that scientists would focus their efforts on precopulatory techniques in which the Y-bearing sperm could be separated from the X-bearing sperm. Early endeavors included centrifuging the sperm suspension at high speeds, placing the sperm suspension in an electrical field (electrophoresis), and treating sperm cells with an antibody to the Y chromosome.[9] None of these early trials yielded unequivocal results. In recent years, Ronald Ericsson of Gametrics Limited of Sausalito, California discovered that liquid albumin, a protein constituent of blood, has a viscosity that apparently is ideal for separating sperm cells.[10] In particular, albumin is thick enough to impede slow moving sperm but sufficiently thin not to hinder fast moving sperm. When semen is placed on top of a column of serum albumin, the sperm cells that filter to the bottom of the column are found to be predominantly Y-bearing sperm. Specifically, eighty percent of the sperm at the bottom have a Y chromosome compared with forty to fifty percent in a random sample of the initial sperm suspension.

Ericsson's success in separating X-bearing and Y-bearing sperm was judged by staining the rapidly moving Y sperm with the flourescent dye (quinacrine mustard).[11] Quinacrine staining of human chromosomes causes

---

[7]R. Guerrero, "Association of the Type and Time of Insemination within the Menstrual Cycle with the Human Sex Ratio at Birth," *New England Journal of Medicine* 291 (1974): 1056-59.

[8]W. H. James, "Time of Fertilization and Sex of Infants," *Lancet* 1 (1980): 1124-26; J. T. France, F. M. Graham, L. Gosling, and P. I. Hair, "A Prospective Study of the Preselection of the Sex of Offspring by Timing Intercourse Relative to Ovulation," *Fertility and Sterility* 41 (1984): 894-900.

[9]M. J. Gordon, "The Control of Sex," *Scientific American* 199, 5 (1958): 87-94; P. Lindahl, "Separation of Bull Spermatozoa Carrying X and Y Chromosomes by Counter-streaming Centrifugation," *Nature* 181 (1958): 784-85.

[10]R. J. Ericsson, C. N. Langevin, and M. Nishino, "Isolation of Fractions Rich in Human Y Sperm," *Nature* 246 (1973); 421-24.

[11]L. Zech, "Investigation of Metaphase Chromosomes with DNA-Binding Fluorochromes," *Experimental Cell Research* 58 (1969): 463.

an intense bright fluorescence of the long arm of the Y chromosome. When sperm cells are treated with quinacrine mustard, the bright fluorescence appears in sperm heads containing the Y chromosome but not in X-bearing sperm. For the first time, an objective method exists of differentiating between Y-bearing and X-bearing sperm.[12] Unfortunately, the stained sperm cannot be retrieved for artificial insemination.

Ericsson's technique has moved from the laboratory to clinical practice. Preliminary results on slightly more than 100 human births following insemination with sperm separated by the Ericsson method have revealed a seventy-seven percent male predominance. The results are promising, but the technology is imperfect. The goal is to refine the technique so that the normal ratio of fifty male: fifty female is modified to 100 male: zero female or, conversely, zero male: 100 female. There are also perplexing findings that presently defy explanation. Among the inexplicable data is the reversal of effect when Clomid-treated women are inseminated with sperm processed by Ericsson's albumin separation technique.[13] When albumin-separated sperm was used in women whose pregnancies were not induced with Clomid, a high proportion of males were delivered. However, when Clomid-teated women were inseminated with albumin-separated sperm, eighty percent had female offspring. This reversal of effect was wholly unexpected.

Researchers remain cautious when appraising the effectiveness of sex preselection technology. Since it is unlikely that viable sperm will be perfectly sexed in the reasonably near future,[14] parents have resorted to amniocentesis to make sex choices. The option of abortion on the basis of sex

---

[12]Although generally accepted that the fluorescent bright spots in sperm after quinacrine staining represent the Y chromosome, there are still some unaccountable findings. Sperm possessing two bright spots would signify the presence of the two Y chromosomes. As high as 5.6 percent of sperm contain two spots, which would be indicative of an exceptionally high nondisjunction rate for the human Y chromosome. Other cytogentic studies of human sperm do not confirm such an elevated nondisjunction frequency. See R. H. Martin, W. Balkan, K. Burns, A. W. Rademaker, C. C. Lin, and N. L. Rudd, "The Chromosome Constitution of 1,000 Human Spermatozoa, *Human Genetics* 63 (1983): 305-309.

[13]F. J. Beernink and R. J. Ericsson, "Male Sex Preselection through Sperm Isolation," *Fertility and Sterility* 38 (1982): 493-95.

[14]The unequivocal separation of the Y-bearing sperm from the X-bearing sperm may be closer at hand than here envisioned. It may be that hybridization probes for DNA sequences specific to the X or Y chromosomes will be available in the reasonably near future.

has become a stark reality. Indeed, the stratagem used by some couples to achieve a balanced family composition could easily be regarded as duplicity.[15] In one instance, a pregnant thirty-eight-year-old woman, who already had one boy and two girls, requested amniocentesis ostensibly to rule out Down syndrome. Karyotype analysis revealed a chromosomally normal female. The woman then sought an abortion since she and her husband desired another son. Since many physicians believe that sex choice is not a compelling reason for abortion, some hospitals have opted to withhold prenatal information on the sex of the fetus unless it is critical for the management of the pregnancy. But to block access to information about the fetus is to deny the right of the woman to make a decision about abortion that remains hers to make, legally at least.

Although sex choice by amniocentesis is effective, it is vehemently controversial. Some authors have been inclined to condone sex selection on the grounds of the woman's right to decide the disposition of her pregnancy.[16] In acknowledging the woman's right to self-determination, the Supreme Court largely acted on behalf of women with unwanted pregnancies who had been confronted with legal barriers to abortion.[17] In such a context, one can understand the basis for the woman's right to control her reproduction. However, the context is assuredly different when amniocentesis is contemplated for fetal-sex determination. In this circumstance, the woman is not faced with an unwanted pregnancy but rather has knowingly undertaken childbearing. To endorse a prospective mother seeking amniocentesis for the sole reason of sex selection, with the possible consequence of certain death for the fetus if the sex is inappropriate, is to sanction what many consider an unacceptable understanding of what having a family means.

---

[15]M. A. Stenchever, "An Abuse of Prenatal Diagnosis," *Journal American Medical Association* 221 (1972): 408; G. A. Dove and C. Blow, "Boy or Girl Parental Choice?" *British Medical Journal* 2 (1979): 1399-1400.

[16]J. C. Fletcher, "Ethics and Amniocentesis for Fetal Sex Identification," *New England Journal Medicine* 301 (1979): 550-53. In this article, Fletcher espouses the principle of reproductive freedom, and supports the concept of fetal sexing for family planning. In a later article, Fletcher re-examines his view and reverses his early position by stating that sex selection is an unethical practice. See J. C. Fletcher, "Is Sex Selection Ethical?" In *Research Ethics* (New York: Alan R. Liss, Inc., 1983) 333-48.

[17]*Roe v. Wade* and *Doe v. Bolton*. U.S. Supreme Court Reports, 35 L. Ed. 2d (1973): 147-222.

Physicians almost universally believe that the termination of pregnancy must rest on medical grounds. But the physician may be placed in an uncomfortable position if he or she dismisses sex choice as "trivial." After all, medicine often treats desires rather than needs. Accordingly, it has been argued by some that the physician should accommodate the woman's wishes with respect to sex selection. Perhaps the most cogent argument against conceiving a child with the view of choosing a particular sex is that the course of action represents the pinnacle of sex discrimination. To condone sex choice—whether it be for a male or a female child—would imply that the worth of a human being rests on its gender.[18]

---

[18]Parents who are at risk for transmitting a sex-linked hereditary disorder have reasonable justification for requesting fetal sex identification. Approximately 200 sex-linked diseases have been described, including hemophilia, muscular dystrophy, and Lesch-Nylan syndrome. Sex selection represents the most accessible and reliable method for the avoidance of severe sex-linked disorders.

Chapter 10

Clones and Chimeras

In 1978, the free-lance writer David Rorvik, promoted his book entitled *In His Image: The Cloning of a Man.*[1] Rorvik made the extravagant claim that a genetically identical replica, or clone, had been created of an eccentric, aging millionaire. Presumably, in September 1973, a sixty-seven-year-old millionaire named ''Max'' asked Rorvik for help in arranging the cloning of an heir. Rorvik wrote that he introduced Max to a scientist named ''Darwin,'' who agreed to undertake the project at a secret laboratory set up outside the United States and totally financed by the millionaire. Then, in March 1975, Darwin reportedly was able to incorporate a body cell taken from Max into a human egg from which the nucleus had been removed. The resulting embryo was implanted in the uterus of a sixteen-year-old virgin, who gave birth to a boy alleged to be an exact genetic copy of Max. Rorvik's book was rushed into print three months ahead of schedule, so that this incredible story could be foisted early on a naive public.

All members of the scientific community viewed with astonishment the readiness with which the general public and news media accepted the bold assertions by Rorvik. The popular press contributed its usual brand of exaggeration with stories of cloning that were more startling than enlight-

---

[1]D. M. Rorvik, *In his Image: The Cloning of Man* (Philadelphia: J. B. Lippincott Company, 1978).

ening. Any knowledgeable person familiar with the available techniques and current findings on cloning would have immediately dismissed Rorvik's claims as blatantly impossible. Yet, it took a congressional hearing and the sober testimony of several respected scientists to impress upon the average citizen that the claims of a cloned human was pure fiction and a hoax.[2]

Theoretically, the production of an exact copy, or genetic replica, of a human being is one of the more startling possibilities of the new reproductive technologies. An individual may be able to confer immortality on himself or herself simply by giving up a few of his or her body cells. In other words, a person in one generation can prepare an additional copy of himself or herself for another trial in the next generation. Indeed, a person may place a few cells in cold storage, with the flattering (or grim) prospect that his or her cells might be cloned several generations later. The cloned individual is, in reality, not an offspring; it is its own parent reincarnated in new cytoplasm. But all this still remains in the realm of the highly theoretical.

Extravagant claims of the popular press serve only to contribute to the already distorted public view of the aspirations and accomplishments of scientists. Sensational pronouncements have greater news value than sober statements of fact, and for this reason news concerning science and technology often appears embroidered. Actually, most scientists have restrained thoughts concerning the possibility of the deliberate production of genetic copies of humans. In fact, the scientific community dismisses the application of cloning techniques to humans as the blue-sky ramblings of a handful of imaginative investigators and flamboyant journalists.

It is important to appreciate how the investigations on cloning were originally conceived and conducted. Cloning experiments were first undertaken on frogs in the 1950s by Drs. Robert Briggs and Tom King, both then at the Institute for Cancer Research in Philadelphia.[3] Their aim was

---

[2]"Developments in Cell Biology and Genetics: Hearing before the Subcommittee on Health and the Environment of the Committee on Interstate and Foreign Commerce, House of Representatives," *Developments,* Serial No. 95-105 (31 May 1978; Washington DC: U.S. Government Printing Office).

[3]The pioneer work by Briggs and King as well as subsequent studies by other investigators are aptly reviewed by R. G. McKinnell, *Cloning: A Biologist Reports.* (Minneapolis: University of Minnesota Press, 1979). See also J. B. Gurdon, "Transplanted Nuclei and Cell Differentiation," *Scientific American* 219 (1968): 24-35.

to determine whether a nucleus from a cell of an embryo could actually cause an egg, deprived of its nucleus, to develop. Experimentally, they succeeded in removing the nucleus of an unfertilized frog egg and replacing it with a nucleus from one of the cells of a developing frog embryo.

The experimental design is shown in figure 15. The recipient unfertilized egg is first stimulated, or activated, with a sharp fine needle. This activation causes the egg to rotate so that the nucleus is uppermost. The egg nucleus, which now lies just under the surface of the egg, is removed by placing a glass needle directly beneath the nucleus and then pulling the needle up through the egg surface. The small mass of cytoplasm lifted out contains the egg nucleus.

The next step is to replace the egg nucleus that has been removed with one that has been obtained from a developing donor embryo (technically, a blastula). A prospective donor cell is taken from a blastula that has been dissociated (that is separated into individual cells) in a special solution. The donor cell is carefully drawn up in a micropipette and then injected into the previously enucleated recipient egg.

The remarkable finding was that an enucleated egg injected with a nucleus from an advanced embryo can develop into a normal frog. In essence, a nucleus from an embryo can promote normal development of an egg, thereby bypassing the usual process of fertilization of egg by sperm. This process may be repeated (say, three times, as illustrated in figure 15) to produce several genetically identical individuals or, technically, a clone. The work is exceedingly important from a purely scientific standpoint, since it shows that an embryonic cell, not merely the sperm and egg, contains all the necessary information to create a new individual.

No scientist has undertaken, or has even seriously contemplated, the transplantation of the nucleus of a human embryonic cell (or adult cell) into a human egg. The fact that such experimentation in humans is unthinkable or uninviting is no basis for rejecting investigations of this type in other mammalian species. Indeed, successful nuclear transplantation has recently been achieved in a mammal—the mouse. The cloning of mice was performed at the University of Geneva, Switzerland by Dr. Karl Illmensee of that institution in collaboration with Dr. Peter Hoppe of the Jackson Laboratory in Bar Harbor, Maine.[4] The two investigators transplanted a

---

[4]K. Illmensee and P. C. Hoppe, "Nuclear Transplantation in Mus Musculus: Developmental Potential of Nuclei from Preimplantation Embryos," *Cell* 23 (1981): 9-18.

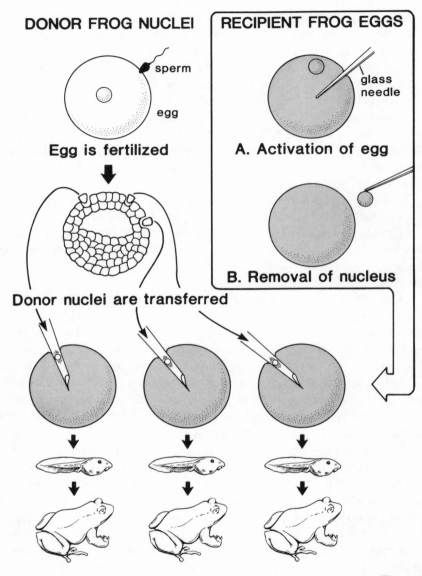

Cloning of a Frog

Figure 15

When three cells from a single embryo are injected individually into enucleated eggs, the three recipient eggs develop into genetically identical individuals ("triplets").

nucleus extracted from a seven-day-old mouse embryo into a recently fertilized mouse egg whose own nuclear material had been removed (figure 16).[5] The donor nucleus came from the embryonic cell of a gray strain of mouse, whereas the recipient egg was derived from a black strain. The recipient egg was then cultured *in vitro* to the blastocyst stage, at which time it was placed in the uterus of a foster female of a white strain. At term, the newborn possessed a gray coat, signifying that the genetic information in the transplanted donor nucleus governed development. Stated differently, the newborn did not show characteristics of the black strain which furnished the original fertilized egg, nor traits of the white foster mother in which gestation occurred.[6]

Despite the accomplishment in the mouse, progress with mammals has been slow because of the many technical difficulties in working with mammalian eggs (including human eggs). Mammalian eggs are produced in relatively few numbers and are much more fragile than frog eggs. Moreover, frog eggs are normally fertilized and develop outside the female body, whereas mammalian eggs must be grown in culture until they reach the stage at which they can implant in the uterus. The task has been made easier with the advent of *in vitro* fertilization. But even with the *in vitro* capabilities, it would be extremely difficult to justify cloning in humans, if only because of the low success rate in both the frog and the mouse. In mice experiments, only one out of seven transplanted nuclei promotes development, and not all of the resulting embryos are normal.[7]

---

[5]In the experiment by Illmensee and Hoppe, the donor nucleus was taken from the "inner cell mass" of a mouse blastocyst. In mammalian development, the inner cell mass is the embryo proper that develops into the fetus. The remaining cells that surround the inner cell mass as a circular layer (see figure 4 above) constitute the "trophoblast," which gives rise to the structures (e.g., chorion and allantois) required for maintenance and nourishment of the fetus.

[6]To date, the fascinating experiments by Illmensee and Hoppe have not been repeated in another laboratory. Generally, outstanding scientific research is verified by other investigators using the same methods. (See J. L. Marx, "Bar Harbor Investigation Reveals No Fraud," *Science* 220 [1983]: 1254; C. Norman, "No Fraud Found in Swiss Study," *Science* 223 [1983]: 913).

[7]It should be underscored that only embryonic cells have the capacity to direct an enucleated egg to develop. The cells of an adult individual are so differentiated that they have lost this unique ability. Hence, it would be almost impossible to create a human clone from an existing adult individual, as Rorvik claimed in his outrageous book (see n. 1).

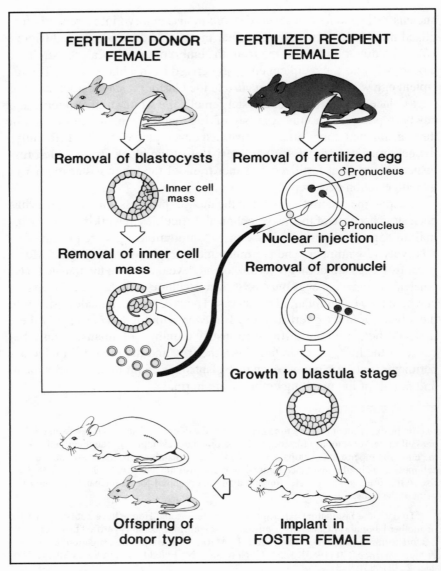

Cloning of a Mouse   **Figure 16**

A cell from one mouse embryo (donor) can be transferred into an enucleated egg of another strain (recipient), and then grown in a foster female of a third strain. The resulting offspring displays traits of the original donor, and has no characteristics of strains provided by the recipient egg or foster mother.

We do know that the early cells of mammalian embryos are "totipotent"—that is, that each cell in the early embryo has the ability to develop into a whole, complete embryo.[8] Thus, if one were to disjoin the two cells after the fertilized egg had divided, each of the two isolated cells would not develop into half of an organism, but rather into two normal and complete individuals (in fact, identical twins).[9] The finding that the mammalian egg has a plastic organization has received striking confirmation in the remarkable studies by Dr. Beatrice Mintz of the Cancer Institute in Philadelphia.[10] Rather than separate the two-cell stage to produce identical twins, Mintz merged, or fused, the cleavage cells derived from two different mouse embryos (figure 17). The composite embryo is sometimes referred to as a *chimera,* since it contains the tissues of two distinct genetic types.[11]

In this operation, the tough membrane surrounding the embryo (technically, the *zona pellucida*) is disrupted, or dissolved, by a protein-splitting enzyme. The two denuded embyos are placed in contact in a culture medium. The cells from each embryo unite to form a composite sphere that

---

[8]The individual cells of the early (cleaving) mammalian embryo are highly "labile" or "plastic" in the sense that a given cell is *not* predetermined to form particular structures or organs. In fact, even if all but one cell in a two-celled, four-celled, or eight-celled embryo were removed, the remaining one cell is capable of developing into a normal full-term fetus. (See A. K. Tarkowski, "Experiments in the Development of Isolated Blastomeres of Mouse Eggs," *Nature* 184 [1959]: 1286-87; N. W. Moore, C. Adams, and L. E. A. Rowson, "Developmental Potential of Single Blastomeres of the Rabbit Egg," *Journal of Reproduction and Fertility* 17 (1968): 527-31.

[9]The manipulative technology is so highly developed and sophisticated that reproductive biologists today can artificially cleave a single mammalian fertilized egg into two, and each separated half can be implanted in a separate foster mother. At Colorado State University, two genetically identical colts were born in 1984 by this procedure, each having been carried by a separate brood mare. See G. Maranto, "Clones on the Range," *Discover* 5(1984): 34-38.

[10]B. Mintz, "Gene Control of Mammalian Pigmentary Differentiation. 1. Clonal Origin of Melanocytes," *Proceedings of the National Academy of Science* 58(1967): 344-51.

[11]In Greek mythology, the classical chimera was composed of three parts—a lion's head, a goat's body, and a serpent's tail. Incredulous as it may seem, modern investigators have experimentally created viable chimeras composed of two parts—a sheep and a goat. See C. B. Fehilly, S. M. Willadsen and E. M. Tucker, "Interspecific Chimaerism between Sheep and Goat," *Nature* 307 (1984): 634-36; S. Meinecke-Tillmann and B. Meinecke, "Experimental Chimeras—Removal of Reproductive Barrier between Sheep and Goat," *Nature* 307(1984): 637-38.

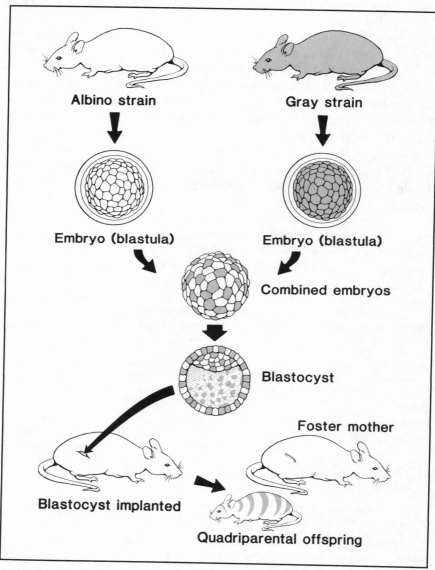

Albino strain

Gray strain

Embryo (blastula)

Embryo (blastula)

Combined embryos

Blastocyst

Foster mother

Blastocyst implanted

Quadriparental offspring

Chimerism

Figure 17

The formation of a chimeric blastocyst by the fusion of two embryos (blastulae) derived from two different mouse strains. Since the resulting single chimeric offspring has four parents, it is often referred to as a quadriparental offspring.

becomes a single blastocyst. This chimeric embryo is then surgically transplanted in the uterus of a foster mother, where it develops normally. Many of these embryos have grown into healthy, breeding adults. The first viable chimeric mouse was born in 1965. Since then, some 1,000 normal animals have been experimentally produced, and many lived out a full life span. They, in turn, have left over 25,000 offspring.

Evidently, the mammalian fertilized egg, as well as the early cleavage cells, do not have fixed fates restricted to an indelible course of development. The cells of the early developmental stages have great plasticity. The ease of experimental manipulation of the early embryonic cells has proved invaluable in another series of intriguing experiments, which may have great practical consequences. It is well known that a tissue or organ transplanted from one individual to another genetically different individual provokes an immune response by the recipient. The grafted tissue or organ is typically destroyed because the host recognizes the graft as foreign and mounts destructive substances (antibodies) against it. Accordingly, unless the host antibody response is suppressed in some way, it can be expected that any foreign transplanted material will not be permanently accepted by the host. In the 1950s, the English biologist Peter Medawar and his colleagues discovered a unique way of overcoming rejection of a foreign graft.[12]

Medawar found that foreign cells introduced into the *embryonic* period of the host would be treated by the host as if it were its own cells. In other words, the host will fail to react against any of the donor cells with which it would come into contact in later (adult) life. It is as if the host had been deceived by the artificial introduction of the alien cells early in life and had learned to recognize these alien cells on its own. As illustrated in figure 18, cells from one embryo (donor blastocyst) can be transferred to another embryo (host blastocyst).[13] In adult life, a piece of skin (which ordinarily would be rejected) can be successfully grafted from the donor animal to

---

[12]P. B. Medawar, "Immunological Tolerance," *Science* 133 (1961): 303-306; F. M. Burnet, "The Mechanism of Immunity," *Scientific American* 204 (1961): 58-67.

[13]The experiments described are based on investigations by the reproductive physiologist R. L. Gardner of Cambridge University. See R. L. Gardner, "Mouse Chimeras Obtained by the Injection of Cells into the Blastocyst," *Nature* 220 (1968): 596-97 and R. L. Gardner and M. F. Lyon, "X-Chromosome Inactivation Studies by Injection of a Single Cell into a Mouse Blastocyst." *Nature* 231 (1971): 385-86.

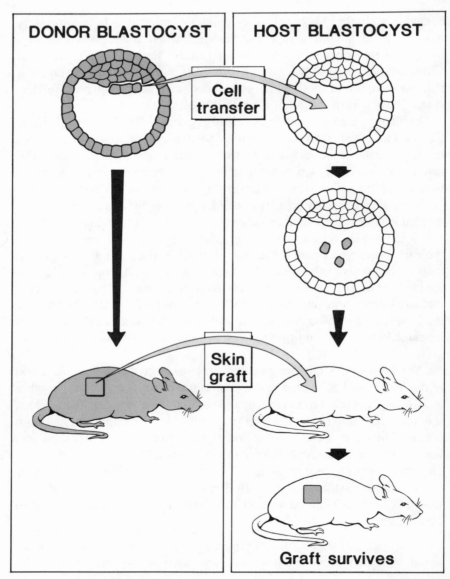

Induction of Immunological Tolerance   **Figure 18**

Cells taken from the embryo (blastocyst) of one mouse strain (donor) are injected into the cavity of a blastocyst of another mouse strain (host). When the host becomes an adult, it readily accepts (tolerates) a skin graft from the donor-strain adult.

the host animal. The host can now receive a variety of grafts tissue from the donor, including a liver, spleen, kidney, and bone marrow. Thus, an organism exposed to a foreign cell in an early developmental stage fails to develop the capacity to respond immunologically to that foreign cell if introduced again in adult life. For having arrived at this important concept known as "immunological tolerance," Peter Medawar was one of the recipients of the 1960 Nobel Prize in Physiology or Medicine.

One might wonder whether the foregoing phenomenon of immunological tolerance would ever have practical applicability in humans. The experimentation in mice has not been extended to humans, but the basic, underlying principles have been brought to bear in a real-life situation.[14] The bizarre episode involves a wife's deliberate plan to provide her ailing husband with the kidneys of a fetus intentionally conceived and aborted to save her husband's life. A twenty-eight-year-old male engineer has suffered from kidney damage and has been on dialysis for several years. His ailment and time-consuming therapy have precluded any meaningful employment. An unusual blood type has limited his chances of a kidney transplant from a suitable donor. His wife suggested a way of obtaining a matching donor. She expressed the willingness to become pregnant with the intent of aborting the fetus, at five or six months, to obtain transplantable kidneys. The transplant of fetal kidneys is technically possible, with a good prognosis that the fetal graft would not be rejected by the husband.

Is an intentional abortion for transplantable kidneys defensible by any measure of morality?

---

[14]Factual case studies demonstrating ethical dilemmas in medicine appear regularly in the *Hastings Center Report*. For the particular case presented herein, see M. A. Warren, D. Maguire, and C. Levine, "Can the Fetus Be an Organ Farm?" *Hastings Center Report* 8 (1978): 23-25.

Chapter 11

Doctoring the Genes

There is no effective treatment for most severe genetic disorders. Some, like Tay-Sachs disease, follow a relentless course to early death; others, like Lesch-Nyhan syndrome, are crippling, painful disorders that linger for many years. Debilitating and often fatal inherited disorders are largely caused by coding defects in the gene. In many cases, only one miscoded gene can trigger a major disorder. As a result of a single faulty gene, the body may fail to manufacture an important protein or enzyme. The absence or deficiency of a vital chemical substance may lead to the malfunctioning of several different bodily processes.

When an infant is born with a serious inherited condition, the physician today can do very little in terms of therapy. Existing treatments are more palliative than curative. However, in the years to come, some of the life-threatening genetic disorders may be corrected by a procedure known as *gene therapy*. In theory, the procedure is deceptively simple: a faulty gene is replaced by, or compensated by, a properly functioning gene. In reality, however, the task is formidable. The normal gene must first be isolated from among one or more million human genes; the gene must then be inserted into the appropriate target cells; and the gene, once incorporated, must be able to function properly in its new location without causing harm. Despite numerous impediments, the treatment of human disorders by gene therapy is almost within the grasp of medical scientists.[1]

---

[1]"Gene therapy" is a highly charged emotional expression. The apprehension in the general public is that human genes will be manipulated to remake or change the nature of

Investigators currently can isolate a human gene by taking advantage of the fact that genes are the repositories of information for proteins. Stated another way, a gene is a DNA sequence that directs the production of a specific protein. The gene (DNA) does not directly form a protein but works in a complex way through another large molecule known as "messenger RNA." In carrying manufacturing instructions for the protein from the gene, the messenger RNA molecule is like a photographic negative of the gene. Thus, by "printing" the messenger RNA extracted from a human cell, a copy of the gene is "developed." These copies of human genes are then introduced into bacteria, which divide repeatedly and replicate the human gene innumerable times. Under proper conditions, one bacterial cell can divide into one billion identical cells in the short span of ten hours. Accordingly, the bacterial colony becomes the source of a virtually limitless number of copies of a human gene.

With the isolated human gene on hand, the next step is to insert the gene inside the nucleus of the target cell. Several techniques have been devised, but attention of late has centered on viruses as the most reliable vehicle for transfer.[2] Much of the native genetic information of viruses can be selected, and replaced by the genes of other organisms, including humans.

In 1984, Richard C. Mulligan and his associates at the Massachusetts Institute of Technology "packaged" a virus to transfer an antibiotic-resistant gene from a particular strain of bacteria to bone marrow tissue of a

---

human beings, like Dr. Frankenstein's monster. The public fears the exercise of inordinate power by scientists. Such anxiety is misplaced, reflecting in large measure the public's lack of understanding of the motivations and goals of scientists. The objective of biomedical research is, and has always been, to alleviate human suffering. The focus of gene therapy is on debilitating, rare inherited disorders caused by simple mutations. Even when the techniques become perfected, only a few of the 3,000 known single-gene disorders are likely to be treatable. Gross traits like personality, intelligence, and physical prowess are controlled or influenced by such large numbers of genes that their deliberate modification is not amenable, now or in the foreseeable future, to the tools of gene therapy.

[2]Viruses known as retroviruses are uniquely suited for the role of transferring genes because, unlike most other viruses, they do not destroy the host cell. Moreover, retroviruses normally insert their own viral genes into the chromosomes of the host. In other words, retroviruses cannot themselves survive or reproduce unless they become incorporated in the nuclear DNA of the host.

mouse.[3] The targets for gene insertion were the blood-forming stem cells, a population of precursor cells from which adult blood cells are derived. These stem cells comprise less than 0.1 percent of marrow tissue. If the stem cells were to incorporate the antibiotic-resistant gene introduced by the engineered viruses, then the recipient mouse would possess the bacterial gene in every type of differentiated blood cell derived from the stem cells carrying the implanted gene. In conformity with exception, the antibiotic-resistant gene was found to be present in differentiated white blood cells of the spleen. This finding was clear-cut evidence of successful gene transfer since the mature blood cells of the spleen of the recipient mouse could only have originated from the introduced stem cells. The efficiency of gene transfer was only twenty percent—that is, the engineered viruses integrated only in a subpopulation of the stem cells. Moreover, the viruses could not be targeted to particular sites in the chromosomes. Nevertheless, the technology is at hand for removing a small stretch of viral DNA and replacing the deleted region with a normal human gene that can code for the desired product (figure 19).

The immediate hopes for somatic cell therapy in humans revolve around those diseases that can be treated by modifying the blood-forming cells of the bone marrow, since this tissue can be readily removed, manipulated *in vitro,* and easily reintroduced into an intact host. Several heritable immunodeficient disorders are manifested primarily in bone marrow-derived cells, prominent among them purine nucleoside phosphorylase (PNP) deficiency and adenosine deaminase (ADA) deficiency. Both rare disorders are conspicuous by their predisposition to recurrent and persistent infections. ADA deficiency attracted public notice because of David, the remarkable "bubble boy." David, whose last name has been withheld for privacy, died at age twelve in a Houston, Texas hospital on 22 February 1984. David spent all but his last fifteen days in a germ-free plastic bubble.

In ADA deficiency, the failure to produce the appropriate enzyme in purine metabolism causes a marked deficiency of specific blood cells

---

[3]D. A. Williams, I. R. Lemischka, D. G. Nathan, and R. C. Mulligan, "Introduction of New Genetic Material into Pluripotent Haematopoietic Stem Cells of the Mouse," *Nature* 310 (1984): 476-80. See also R. Mann, R. C. Mulligan, and D. Baltimore, "Construction of a Retrovirus Packaging Mutant and Its Use to Produce Helper-Free Defective Retrovirus," *Cell* 33 (1983): 153-59; A. Joyner, G. Keller, R. A. Phillips, and A. Bernstein. "Retrovirus Transfer of a Bacterial Gene into Mouse Haematopoietic Progenitor Cells," *Nature* 305 (1983): 556-58.

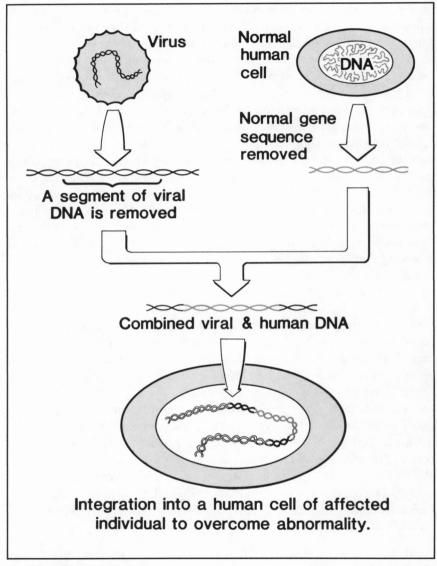

Virus-Mediated Gene Transfer   **Figure 19**

A virus can be engineered to mediate the transfer of a normal human gene into a genetically affected individual to overcome the detrimental effects of the faulty gene.

(lymphocytes) that protect the body against a variety of harmful pathogens. Even the production of a small fraction of the normal enzyme activity (ten to fifteen percent of normal) would be beneficial to the patient. The hope is that enzyme production can be fostered by placing the appropriate normal human gene via a virus into human patients.[4] The protocol calls for removing the defective bone marrow from a patient, inserting a normal enzyme-producing gene into a number of marrow cells, and then reimplanting the treated bone marrow into the patient. Tests with experimental animals have been very promising.[5]

Although the techniques of gene therapy have become increasingly refined, clinical trials in humans await additional studies with laboratory animals to obviate potential risks to the patient. With apologies to our first astronauts, several more small steps in the experimental mouse must be forthcoming before undertaking any giant leap for mankind. There continue to exist great uncertainties about the eventual outcome of transferring a human gene.[6] So far, there is no assurance that the transferred gene will function normally or predictably. The means of programming the virus so that the human gene can be inserted into a specific region of the chromo-

---

[4]R. Parkman, E. W. Gelfand, F. S. Rosen, A. Sanderson, and R. Hirschhorn. "Severe Combined Immunodeficiency and Adenosine Deaminase Deficiency," *New England Journal of Medicine* 292 (1975): 714-19; R. Hirschhorn, V. Roegner-Maniscalco, and L. Kuritsky, "Bone Marrow Transplantation Only Partially Restores Purine Metabolites to Normal in Adenosine Deaminase-Deficient Patients," *Journal of Clinical Investigation* 68 (1981): 1387-93.

[5]Several investigators are vigorously pursuing the viral approach to transferring normal human genes. In another important investigation, Theodore Friedmann and Douglas Jolly of the University of California, in collaboration with Inder Verma and Dusty Miller at the Salk Institution, have placed the human gene for a specific transferase enzyme into retroviruses and have then infected bone marrow cells of laboratory mice with the genetically engineered viruses. In humans, an infant born with a defective gene that fails to code for the specific transferase suffers from Lesch-Nyhan disease, characterized by progressive mental retardation, cerebral palsy, self-mutilation, and the accumulation of uric acid in the body. See A. D. Miller, D. J. Jolly, T. Friedmann, and I. M. Verma, "A Transmissible Retrovirus Expressing Human Hypoxanthine Phosphoribosyltransferase (HPRT): Gene Transfer into Cells Obtained from Humans Deficient in HPRT," *Proceedings of the National Academy of Sciences 80* (1983): 4709-13; A. D. Miller, R. J. Eckner, D. J. Jolly, T. Friedman, and I. M. Verma, "Expression of a Retrovirus Encoding Human HPRT in Mice," *Science* 225 (1984): 630-32.

[6]T. Friedmann, *Gene Therapy: Fact and Fiction in Biology's New Approaches to Disease* (New York: Cold Spring Laboratory, 1983).

some has yet to be devised. The incorporation of the foreign gene in an inappropriate site is potentially dangerous. The improperly inserted gene may alter the function of neighboring genes, producing mutational alterations that can be detrimental to the host.[7] The virus itself may become unstable in its new site and become infectious or virulent. One grim consequence of improper insertion is the activation of cancer-producing genes, known as "oncogenes." There is the possibility that the transferred gene will become located near one of the fifty known oncogenes whose expression could lead to malignancy.[8]

Evidently, before clinical trials in humans are contemplated, it is necessary to weigh the potential risks to the patient, including the possibility of producing a pathologic virus or inducing a cancerous growth, against the anticipated benefits to be gained from the insertion of the functional gene. With crippling and life-threatening disorders, the adverse risks may be low compared to the severity of the disease that might be treatable by gene therapy. In essence, for the foreseeable future, somatic gene therapy is likely to be applied only in rare, specifically chosen genetic disorders.

Most individuals are comfortable with the idea of inserting genetic material in a human patient if the procedure is used for the sole purpose of compensating for malfunctioning genes and overcoming severe genetic defects.[9] In other words, the remedial therapy affects only the treated patient and not later generations. In certain circles, anxieties have surfaced concerning the deliberate genetic modification of the gametes or embryos,

---

[7]E. F. Wagner, L. Covarrubias, T. A. Stewart and B. Mintz, "Prenatal Lethalities in Mice Homozygous for Human Growth Hormone Gene Sequences Integrated in the Germ Line," *Cell* 35 (1983), 647-55; A. Schnieke, K. Harbers and R. Jaenisch, "Embryonic Lethal Mutation Mice Induced by Retrovirus Insertion into the alpha 1 (I) Collagen Gene," *Nature* 304 (1983): 315-20.

[8]The discovery of the existence of oncogenes in human cells is profoundly influencing the direction of cancer research. Oncogenes are genes that, when activated in cells, can transform the cells from normal to cancerous cells. One or more of fifty oncogenes now known to exist normally in human cells can become disruptive to the cells when they become activated to "overexpress" themselves. See J. M. Bishop, "Oncogenes and Proto-Oncogenes," *Hospital Practice* 18 (1983): 67-74; C. M. Croce, "Chromosomal Translocations, Oncogenes, and B-cell Tumors," *Hospital Practice* 20 (1985): 41-48.

[9]J. C. Fletcher, "Moral Problems and Ethical Issues in Prospective Human Gene Therapy," *Virginia Law Review* 69 (1983): 515-46; W. F. Anderson, "Prospects for Human Gene Therapy," *Science* 226 (1984): 401-409.

such that the induced changes are passed on to the offspring.[10] The technique of *in vitro* fertilization has made the embryo accessible to a degree of experimentation not previously possible. In a petri dish, the embryo can be manipulated at a crucial stage when it is normally inaccessible. Indeed, gene therapy on the embryo probably has a greater chance of practical success than treating an adult tissue such as bone marrow. If the gametes could be genetically repaired, then the inherited disorder would not appear in future generations.

The concerns about genetically modifying the embryo are real in that the genetic transformation of certain traits in laboratory animals has already been accomplished by modern DNA technology. Several investigators have reported success in introducing foreign DNA into the germ line of experimental animals, notably mice, by introducing DNA into fertilized eggs.[11] The approach used has been termed "microinjection," since a finely drawn glass pipette injects the desired gene into the nucleus of the cell. The foreign genes that have been injected include those that code for herpes virus thymidine kinase, human interferon, rabbit hemoglobin, growth hormone mouse metallothionein, immunoglobulin, and rat elastase. In many instances, the purified genes introduced into mice at early development are stably integrated and even expressed in the adult host. To cite one report among many, Thomas Wagner and his colleagues[12] transferred by direct microinjection the gene coding for rabbit hemoglobin into the fertilized eggs of mice. The resulting embryos were cultured *in vitro* to the blastocyst stage and then implanted in foster mothers. Not only did the microinjected rabbit gene become integrated into the genetic makeup of the mice that were born, but the rabbit gene was transmitted to the next generation of mice.

Perhaps the most dramatic of the recent reports involves the correction, at least in part, of an hereditary growth deficiency by providing a dwarf

---

[10]C. Grobstein and M. Flower, "Gene Therapy: Proceed with Caution," *Hastings Center Report* 14 (1984): 13-17.

[11]R. D. Palmiter and R. L. Brinster, "Transgenic Mice," *Cell* 41 (1985): 343-65.

[12]T. E. Wagner, P. C. Hoppe, J. D. Jollick, D. R. Scholl, et al., "Microinjection of a Rabbit β-Globin Gene into Adult Mice and Their Offspring," *Proceedings of the National Academy of Sciences* 78 (1981): 6376-80.

mutant mouse with growth hormone by gene therapy.[13] These investigators inserted a normal gene coding for a growth hormone (from a rat) into embryos of a mouse. The embryo evidently had integrated the transplanted growth gene, inasmuch as the newborn were almost double the size of their untreated brothers and sisters. In turn, many of the offspring of the treated individuals retained both the transferred gene and the uncharacteristic large size. Indeed, there were three generations of these "mighty mice."

These pioneering experiments have not been free of troublesome complications. Only about one percent of the inoculated eggs developed into mice that expressed the microinjected gene. Moreover, the newly introduced gene failed to produce the proper amount of the desired product; the gigantism that resulted among the offspring signified that the implanted gene was producing unregulated excessive amounts of growth hormone. Finally, the foreign gene unsuspectedly had adversely affected other characteristics of the animal. In particular, the chronic elevated production of growth hormone had impaired the fertility of the females. All these unfavorable features argue persuasively against applying the present imprecise technology to human embryos.

It has been said that the correction of a genetic disorder by gene therapy on an early embryo might be defensible if there were no alternative, more effective techniques available. Consider sickle cell anemia, an enfeebling single-gene blood disease. This disease can be detected prenatally by analysis of fetal cells of the amniotic fluid (amniocentesis) or fetal cells of the placenta (chorionic villus sampling). Thus, prenatal diagnosis offers the parents the option of terminating the pregnancy if the fetus is demonstrably affected. But not all parents wish to avail themselves of prenatal diagnosis because they are unwilling to accept the option of abortion. Moreover, some genetic disorders, including sickle-cell anemia, may not be judged by the parents to be sufficiently incapacitating to warrant ter-

---

[13]R. D. Palmiter, R. L. Brinster, R. E. Hammer, M. E. Trumbauer, et al. "Dramatic Growth of Mice That Develop from Eggs Microinjected with Metallothionein—Growth Hormone Fusion Genes," *Nature* 300 (1982): 611-15; R. E. Hammer, R. D. Palmiter, and R. L. Brinster, "Partial Correction of Murine Hereditary Growth Disorder by Germ-Line Incorporation of a New Gene," *Nature* 311 (1984): 65-67; and R. D. Palmiter, G. Norstedt, R. E. Gelinas, R. E. Hammer, and R. L. Brinster. "Metallothionein—Human GH Fusion Genes Stimulate Growth of Mice," *Science* 222 (1983): 809-914.

mination of pregnancy. For some parents, then, gene therapy on the gametes or embryo might be the only acceptable, if not efficient, means of preventing the transmission of specific malfunctioning genes to their immediate offspring, as well as future generations. The wish to eliminate the faulty gene once and for all from the family lineage might be very compelling.[14]

---

[14]There are some genetic diseases that may be treatable only by gene therapy on the embryos. Lesch-Nyhan disease falls into this category. The neurological effects are caused by the lack of an enzyme (a specific transferase) in the brain cells. Because of the blood-brain barrier, the brain cells of a Lesch-Nyhan patient would be inaccessible to somatic cells, such as bone marrow cells, that are treated by gene therapy. Early embryonic intervention that affects all cells of the developing individual may be the only means of treating cells or tissues that are not amenable to genetic repair after birth.

Epilogue

When *in vitro* fertilization left the quiet academic halls to become a clinical reality, child-bearing no longer remained a personal and private affair between couples and physicians. Today every facet of reproductive behavior is scrutinized by the widest possible audience. The new reproductive technologies have been the subject of sensational articles by newspapers and magazines. An interested public is now aware, at least in dim outlines, of such dramatic procedures as the freezing of embryos, surrogate motherhood, cloning, and gene therapy. Some people see the new technologies as the fulfillment of a promise by the medical profession to alleviate the anxiety and suffering of childless couples. Others view the medical advances as still another ominous step toward further control and manipulation of basic life processes.

It has been said that the American public has largely remained silent on the profound ethical questions raised by the new reproductive technologies. It has even been suggested that our society has become morally bankrupt. On the contrary, it appears that the public at large has not grown indifferent but has become increasingly tolerant of individual differences. A democratic, pluralistic society seems to be embracing the ideal of *respect for persons*. A central feature of this ideal is that persons are to be treated in ways that respect their freedom of choices. In the context of new reproductive technologies, an individual has the freedom to apply knowledge gained from medical advances to achieve (or avoid) reproduction, while at the same time treating with impartiality those who would not themselves use such freedom. Persons who want to avail themselves of *in vitro* fertilization are free to do so; those who do not are not blameworthy. In essence, each person exercises freedom of choice, and no person's rights are to be compromised in the exercise of a given choice.

Index

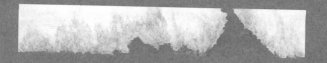